Self-Cured Addict

I Didn't Want Opioids to Kill Me,
So I invented a Device that
Became My Off-Ramp

by

NEIL BRERETON JACKSON

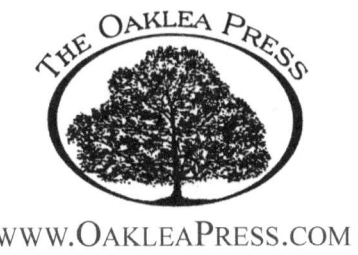

WWW.OAKLEAPRESS.COM

Self-Cured Addict: I Didn't Want Opioids to Kill Me, So I invented a Device that Became My Off-Ramp © 2024 by Neil Brereton Jackson. All rights reserved.

PROPRIETARY RIGHTS: All materials, including without limitation, data or information developed and any ideas, know-how, methodologies, equipment/devices or processes conceived, developed or used or described by above owner; Neil B. Jackson, and N Brereton Medical Technologies, L.L.C., including all USPTO copyrights (c) , trademarks ™ , patents ® , trade secrets and any other proprietary rights related to owner shall be and remain the sole, protected, and exclusive property of owner.

FenBlock is the Registered Trademark of N Brereton Medical Technologies, LLC

DISCLAIMER: The views, opinions, and/or findings are those of the author and should not be construed as an official medical position, policy or decision, unless so designated by other official documentation.

Contents

Foreword 5

PART ONE

Chapter One: Looking Back 9
Chapter Two: The Diagnosis 17
Chapter Three: Radiation Therapy 27
Chapter Four: Prayer Works 31
Chapter Five: Surgery & the Aftermath 35
Chapter Six: Back Home in Lynchburg 40
Chapter Seven: The Wake Up Call 44
    How I Became Free of Hydromorphone
    I Invent a Way to Free Myself from Fentanyl
Chapter Eight: The Cure 57
    Initial Assessment and Customized Plan
    How FenBlock's Barrier Technology Works
    Ongoing Monitoring and Support
    Combining Technology with Medical Oversight
    Getting More Information
Postscript 60
    Reflections

PART TWO

Author's Note 66
Introduction 71
Chapter One: The Scope of the Problem 77
    Prescribed Addiction
    Find Your Courage Through Faith

CONTENTS

Chapter Two: Reflections 112
Chapter Three: Pain & Addiction 125
    Observe, Understand, Accept, Act
Chapter Four: Face the Facts 144
Chapter Five: How C-SPAN Helped 169
Chapter Six: Spreading the Word 178
    My Team, and their impact
Chapter Seven: Overcoming Negativity 184
    Support Groups
Chapter Eight: The Need for a Fentanyl / Opioid Czar .. 201
    Why the End Justifies a New Means
Chapter Nine: Moving Forward 207
    In Conclusion
Afterword 216
Acknowledgements 226
About the Author 236

ADDENDUM

Addiction, Why Is It So Hard to Stop? 238
    Challenging the Status Quo
    Where the Spirit Resides there is Freedom
Youth, Opioids and Gateway Drugs 250
Native American Tribes and Nations 253
The United States Military 255
Departments of Corrections 262
Definitions 266
Types of Pain that are often tied to opioid "relief" 271
Last Page Checklist 274
Letter from Former President Trump 276
Endnotes 277

Foreword

This is the extraordinary and amazing story of Neil Brereton Jackson, a tale that reveals a potential solution to the devastating and deadly scourge of fentanyl addiction that plagues our nation—a true pandemic that took the lives of almost 75,000 Americans in 2023 due to overdoses of that drug.

Besieged with cancer and given a million-to-one chance by his doctor of surviving the surgery that would be required to remove an enormous tumor, Neil experienced what he believes was a message from God telling him that if he survived, he would have an important mission to perform. Miraculously, he survived the surgery, but the mission he anticipated did not materialize immediately. Like many patients given drugs to alleviate severe post-surgical pain, Neil became seemingly hopelessly dependent on opioids.

Seven years passed before his premonition of having a mission came to pass, but it finally did with his invention of FenBlock—a medical device that enables users to break the bond of fentanyl addiction gradually over time while experiencing few if any symptoms of withdrawal.

Self-Cured Addict

It is indeed an honor to publish Neil's story, which I sincerely hope will get the word out about FenBlock with the result that thousands, perhaps even hundreds of thousands of lives will be saved.

    Stephen Hawley Martin
    Editor & Publisher
    The Oaklea Press Inc.

Part One: My Story

As we begin our discussion and story it is a good Time for Reverence

Dear God, as a I come to you weighed down with opioid addiction I pray:

For inner strength and guidance that I may regain
my freedom from addiction and use with Your help.
That You will empower me to manage reducing my use of
their poison and lift up my faith, family, friends and return my health
I pray to You grateful for giving me life, freedom and virtue.
To helping me be an overcomer, to succeed, to bless You
through my work for others.
I will stir myself up today and every day to fight
my addiction with your POWERFUL Armor!
In Jesus' name,

AMEN!

Chapter One: Looking Back

I'm Neil Jackson, a middle class ordinary guy from Barrington, a small working class town in southern New Jersey, right off of Exit 3 of the New Jersey Turnpike, a point of reference understood by New Jerseyans, and this is my story of God's extraordinary use of my life to trust in a higher purpose, to act with faith and humility, and to serve others with love and compassion.

Let me say, however, that I didn't always believe my life had a higher purpose, or that I was here on earth to carry out a mission. That thought came to me at the moment I was diagnosed with a rare form of cancer—cancer that very likely could be fatal. When you're living your life, what happens seems totally random and chaotic. Good things happen, bad things happen—or at least what seem like bad things. As you will soon see, sometimes what appears to be bad, in the end turns out to be good. Now, at age 75, looking back at my life, it appears that events unfolded according to a plan—things happened, people came into my life at specific times, and what the famous psychiatrist Carl Jung called synchronicities occurred—meaningful coincidences that seem to have no logical cause. Rather than chaotic, my life looks more like the plot of a novel written by a bestselling author.

Self-Cured Addict

Let me give you a couple of examples.

What likely caused the illness that brought about that horrific diagnosis was something I had as a kid. I was operated on perhaps six times due to osteochondroma, a cartilage problem in the joints that was benign. I spent a lot of time in the hospital during summer break as a result. I'd be operated on when school let out and then would spend the rest of the summer in recovery before returning to school. That happened several times. Anyway, I later learned that osteochondroma is often the precursor to chondrosarcoma, which is the type of cancer I was diagnosed with later on. But that's not the point I want to make. The point is that what seems like a bad thing, can turn out to be a good thing.

Osteochondroma causes tumors to grow around the joints on the arms and legs, which is not just annoying, the doctors believed those tumors could become malignant if they got banged up and injured. So, as long as they were not in the growth bone area, a surgeon would take them off. Well, a tumor that was taken off my right knee turned out to have been in the growth bone area, and the result was that my leg started to go crooked. Because the bone was weak, my leg went crooked at the knee, and I ended up having to have drastic surgery. The surgeon had to cut into the bone and bend it back so that I could walk properly.

Self-Cured Addict

That was behind me by the time, following high school, I attended Northeastern Christian College. I became active in activities there, and took my studies seriously, but it wasn't long before I realized that preaching was not my calling. Almost immediately after dropping out, good ole President Lyndon Johnson sent me a letter. Apparently, I'd won a free, all expenses paid trip—which could very easily be one way—to Vietnam.

Actually, he sent me two letters. The first was to report for a physical, which I did, and the second was, in the event of selection, to be prepared to report for service at Fort Dix. Concerned whether or not my leg would hold up through basic training, I gathered up all the x-rays and documentation about the operation on my knee and took that along with me. It wasn't that I was against the war—I had friends fighting over there.

So I had another physical, met with a doctor and gave him the x-rays. Then I sat down and waited. The clock clicked and clicked, and about 20 minutes prior to induction, he called me into his office.

The doctor said, "We've been reviewing your file and you're going to be rejected for military service." Then he looked me in the eye, and added, "Congratulations!"

I said, "You know, sir, I can do something in the Army, don't you think?"

Self-Cured Addict

He said, "Mr. Jackson, we wouldn't take you if the war was in your backyard, and let me tell you why. Let's say you go through basic training here at Fort Dix or maybe at Fort Hood. And let's say you injure your leg. Then we'd have to pay you for the rest of your life. It's cheaper to send you to Vietnam, kill you, and send your parents $350 to bury you." He smiled. "Do you want a bus ride home or do you want to go to the mess hall first?"

I said, "I'll take the bus straight home."

I left and I went up to an exit sign. A large and tall gentleman of color was standing there. I walked up to him and handed him my file.

He studied it, looked up and said, "Brother Jackson." (His last name happened to be Jackson.) "Brother Jackson, you've been rejected from military service. Congratulations! Here's your ticket home. Have a good life."

The point of this story is that something that seemed pretty awful at the time, osteochondroma and summers in the hospital and recuperating, may have actually saved my life. I didn't think about it at the time, but later, I did. Maybe I was saved—or maybe I survived, you might say—because I had an important mission to perform.

Here's another example. I did not return to college when I got back from my physical. Instead, I went to work for a bank in what was called "bookkeeping" back then—and no wonder. Almost everything was done by hand using pencils, pens, ledgers and adding machines. That seemed odd to me. Computers were being used in other departments, and it seemed they ought to be put to work everywhere possible in order to make things more efficient. So I told my superiors what I thought and they let me take a crack at it.

As was said above, as I look back, my life seems to have unfolded like a novel. I was at the right place at the right time—I had an aptitude for computers and learned to code. As a result, I became a pioneer in the security and privacy aspect of information technology for the banking industry.

But bookkeeping, auditing and computer programming wasn't all I did at that bank. An attractive young woman named Linda worked in my department, and she caught my eye. Let's face it, usually I'm not shy, and so I didn't waste time. One thing led to another, and within a year we were married.

Neither one of us stayed at that bank very long. Word got around about what I was doing in Information Technology, and I received an attractive offer to form the Data Processing Audit function at Dominion Bankshares in Roanoke, Virginia. To make a short story even shorter, it wasn't long before a moving truck pulled up in front of our home in South Jersey to take us to Roanoke—a place she had never seen and that I had not seen much of. She was pregnant at the time, and we had our son Neil Jr. at Community Hospital in Roanoke.

Some time went by, and I got an even better job offer from Central Fidelity Bank in Lynchburg to create a similar function. I took it, and we relocated to that city, which is a little more than an hour's drive east of Roanoke. That's when I started traveling, and one summer I was sent to take a graduate banking course at the University of Wisconsin. I realized something was wrong when I couldn't get my wife on the phone. This was, of course, before everyone had a cell phone. I was living in a dormitory at the University of Wisconsin, and to make a call, I had to use the phone down the hall. Whenever I tried calling home—no answer. So I started wondering what the heck was going on.

The banking course finally ended. I flew home to Lynchburg, disembarked, and guess what? No wife and kid were there to meet me. Walking through the airport, an announcement came over the loudspeaker, "Neil Jackson, please come to the Piedmont Airlines ticket counter."

A man behind that counter handed me an envelope.

"This was left for you," he said.

Self-Cured Addict

It was a note saying the keys are in the car and the car's in the parking lot.

I called a neighbor. "I'm on my way home, and something's wrong. Do you know what's going on?"

The neighbor said, "I don't know, except that I saw people moving out of your house while you were gone."

The long and short of it is that Linda left me and took our son with her.

I soon found out that in Virginia, the rights of a father were basically non-existent at that time at least. When I told a lawyer I wanted to get custody of my son, he said that the state supreme court had ruled that if a child had a mother, a bad mother is better than no mother at all. Well, I was determined to get custody of my son, nevertheless. I shopped around and found the best lawyer in the state of Virginia when it came to child custody, and I hired him and his partners. I had quite a bit of money saved up at that time, and it cost me every penny of it, but I finally did get custody.

So after six weeks, I was fully divorced and had custody of, "A child of tender loving years," which is what the court calls a child under four years of age. I was the first father in Virginia to do so and probably the second in the nation according to a *Wall Street Journal* article about a guy in

Cincinnati who was the first. For the next several years, I spent most of my free time taking care of my son and reestablishing his relationship with his mother. I knew my responsibility was to assure he loved his mother. I'm not a person who harbors the past.

Still working at Fidelity, I happened to notice a beautiful young woman with a gait of a model coming in and out of the building. I found out where she worked, went to my audit director and asked if he could put me on one of the audits in the trust department—which was her department.

Her name was Darlene. I have to say that once I was there in the trust department, I hesitated to approach her due to her overwhelmingly good looks. Plus she had a southern tone to her voice that gave me chills—it sounded so kind. But we finally met and within a year I married this stunning blonde with flowing waist length hair that radiated in any light. Today, 47 years later, I still can't believe my good fortune. We had three wonderful children, a lot of pets, guinea pigs, fish, dogs, cats—our house was nuts and fun. We all traveled the country at every opportunity.

So you see, even an ugly divorce and custody battle can turn out to be a good thing.

Chapter Two: The Diagnosis

I stayed at Central Fidelity Bank until it was acquired by Wachovia in 1998 and rose under the mentorship of a great General Auditor to the position of Senior Vice President Associate Auditor Information Technology. As mentioned in Chapter One, life was good.

Later on, however, when I was in my 60s and working as a consultant, I began to experience discomfort in my lower back and buttocks. Eventually, the problem grew until I could no longer ignore it. I was, for example, unable to remain seated for very long due to the pain that would develop.

After multiple visits to doctors that involved x-rays and scans that failed to reveal the root of the problem, a trip to the University of Virginia Medical Center in Charlottesville to meet orthopedic oncologist Dr. Greg Domson provided an answer—a diagnosis no one would want. The call came when my wife Darlene and I were in the car, in the parking lot of the apartment complex where we lived. We had a ten-year-old grandson Gavin with us.

I put the phone on speaker mode.

Dr. Domson said that he had some bad news and some good news. "It's cancer," he said. "Which would you like to hear first?"

I said, "I'm a guy that likes to get the bad news out of the way quickly." What I didn't say was that the good news isn't going to help me if the bad news is really bad.

He said, "It's cancer and it's very rare. It's chondrosarcoma, and the problem in your case is where it's positioned in your body. It looks to be a growth around the base of your spine up to the middle of your spine. It has encompassed your pelvis totally, and it's wrapped around your left hip, which is a huge problem." He paused for a moment, and then said, "The other bad news is there's not a physician, including myself, who is trained in what's going to have to take place during the surgery. I've never seen anything like this, and there's nobody in the Commonwealth of Virginia, North Carolina, Maryland, or the Washington DC area that has accomplished anything like what will have to be done. There are only two places where I'd refer you, the Mayo Clinic in Rochester, Minnesota or Massachusetts General Hospital, in Boston."

Dr. Domson was silent for a moment, and just as his words began to sink in, he added, "The second problem is that there's not an operating room large enough in this part of the country. There will need to be perhaps two-dozen people in the operating room during the entire operation, which is a huge, strategic problem. There's no operating room in Virginia or the mid-Atlantic big enough, although both the Mayo Clinic and Mass General have them. We need to work on getting you to doctors at those centers that can do what needs to be done. I'd suggest starting with the Mayo Clinic."

A moment of silence passed, and the doctor asked me what I thought about what he'd just said. I could see that Darlene was already in tears and that my grandson was clearly shocked and about to cry.

I said, "I didn't hear any bad news."

He responded, "You didn't hear any bad news?"

At one time, back when I graduated from high school, I thought I wanted to be a Presbyterian minister, and I went to Northeastern Christian College with that goal. Based on my studies and extracurricular activities, I soon learned, however, that the Church can be very political, with people undercutting each other and jockeying for position. That realization was a big turnoff to me, and so I abandoned the goal of going into the clergy. As a result, my faith was probably comparable to that of most nominal Christians—in other words, nothing out of the ordinary. Until I got the phone call from Dr. Domson and I heard the diagnosis, I had no idea how I would respond. I hadn't prepared myself. Nevertheless, something in me caused me to say, "You know, Dr. Domson, I don't know where this is coming from, but if I'm fortunate enough to come out of the other side of this, I believe God will have a mission and a purpose for me. I don't want to put anything in your hands that you can't handle, but I'm fine."

Self-Cured Addict

At the time, I didn't know what the risk of survival was. That's something I learned about later.

Dr. Domson and I contacted the chief of orthopedic surgery at Mayo Clinic, and we didn't have any problem getting in. That was in January of 2012. We were scheduled for surgery on Valentine's Day, February 14th.

After interviewing the doctor, when I was preparing to go to Minneapolis, I have to say, I had an uneasy feeling that would not go away. Something about the doctor just never settled in my gut. I guess it had to do with the conversation I'd had with him. His "standard plan" was to remove the cancer and my left leg and hip and shift my right leg to be centered under my spine. This all sounded very strange since he had not seen me personally nor obtained any images based on his needs from Mayo Clinic. I didn't want to end up looking like a standing question mark.

I'd asked, "What's your background? How did you get to be an accomplished orthopedic surgeon specializing in a condition so rare as chondrosarcoma?"

He said, "I began my career as a civil engineer, then I changed and went into medicine."

I said, "What's your experience with this type of cancer?"

"I've had five surgeries on chondrosarcoma patients."

Self-Cured Addict

I didn't know whether I was talking to a guy with the most experience or not, and so I said, "What's your success rate?"

He said, "Two are living. One withdrew from the program, and the other two are deceased."

So I thought, *I see. I'm gonna make it fifty-fifty. I'll make six patients, and it'll be three dead or three living.* I also thought his training as an engineer may be a problem when he would face unplanned challenges during surgery. I felt there was an absence of entrepreneurship in his spirit. I was concerned that he may likely turn to technical manuals rather than his gut to fix a problem, thus losing time by being too cautious. I needed an "on the fly fixer" with courage.

Anyhow, I thought about that, and one Thursday morning at three a.m. I woke up with the strong feeling that I know it was God speaking to me; I needed to cancel that appointment and check out Mass General. I got up right then and went to work.

I found a man named Francis Hornicek through the National Institutes of Health who was the number one orthopedic oncologist on chondrosarcoma in the world. I tried to find his email address and found it was protected. But I kept looking, and found lectures and papers he'd written—it was embedded in one of those. I tested it, and it didn't come back, which meant I had a hit. So I wrote to him.

His scheduler called and said they'd received my email, and that in order to become a patient, the doctor had to see me.

Jokingly, I said, "I can't come. I'm in the hills of the western part of Virginia. I don't have any shoes, and the buses don't come through here very often."

She said, "I don't think he's going to change his mind."

I said, "Please ask him again, and I'll send him another email."

So I did, and she asked him again.

The next day, she called me, and said Dr. Hornicek still wants you to come before he accepts you as a patient.

I said, "You're asking an awful lot. I said, it's a thirteen or fourteen hour trip. It will cost a lot of money—what's my rate of return on that?" I thought for a moment and then said, "I'm going to say this—no, I'm not coming. I'll write him one last email."

So I wrote another email. It was on a Thursday. I pleaded with him, and I told him I could get all the data from the orthopedic surgeon at the University of Virginia, that I could have it packaged and sent to him so that he could evaluate it. He was going to have to look at it, anyway, to make his decision.

The last sentence of that email was, "I pray to God that you will accept this."

Self-Cured Addict

It was the craziest thing. Twenty minutes later the phone rang and it was the scheduler. She said Dr. Hornicek wanted to know if I could be there on Monday morning.

I said, "What time?"

She said, "Seven a.m. in the hospital."

I said, "I'll be there."

She said, "We're going to set you up with a concierge service that will help take care of your room." She added, "The American Cancer Society has a program for people traveling for cancer treatment, which enables us to provide you with an American Express travel card. You can use it on this trip or on a future trip. It's on its way."

As it turned out, they put us at the Westin Copley Place. I'd been there on business a number of times, and it is a exceptionally nice hotel.

When we checked in, the desk clerk said, "Oh, I see. You're here for Mass General."

I said, "Right."

He said, "We have a really nice room for you."

They gave us the top floor suite—probably a thousand-dollar-a-night room, overlooking Boston Common: America's oldest public park, with open green spaces, walking paths, and monuments.. It really was really special. A Special thanks to Westin for such kindness, a reflection I would learn is standard at Mass General and almost everywhere cancer is diagnosed or treated.

We got up at 4 a.m. the next morning and arrived at the hospital by seven. Before we met with Dr. Hornicek I had to drink quite a lot of fluid before the CT scan that had been scheduled because this type of cancer is not detectable by a normal x-ray. It's soft tissue that an x-ray doesn't reflect on. I also had to have a couple tattoos so that in the upcoming radiation therapy, they'd be able to line up the equipment properly. They were planning ahead.

Then we were taken to a circular room where doctors in their typically long-sleeved, knee-length white coats were sitting surrounded by computer screens that displayed the images I'd sent overnight on Thursday—this was the following Monday. Suffice it to say they were very well prepared. Everyone in that room knew everything he or she wanted or needed to know about my condition. They were top-notch people, and all of them were very personable. They were cordial to me and to Darlene, and they asked a lot of questions—not of me, but of Dr. Hornicek. Darlene and I came away extremely impressed.

As the meeting wrapped up, Dr. Hornicek explained what the schedule would be. I'd be coming back in March for Proton-Photon radiation treatment that would kill the marginal cells around the tumor.

He said, "The tumor has to come out in one piece. If any living tissue particles from the tumor fall off into your body cavity, you'll be dead in 30 days. So we're going to kill the margins—at least to a certain depth. It'll take six weeks of radiation sessions every day to do it. You may have blisters coming out of your inner skin because it's so intense.

Dr. Hornicek then turned from me to address his colleagues and said, "Before Mr. and Mrs. Jackson leave, I want to reiterate what I said to him earlier, and I want you to hear what he says. I told Mr. Jackson he had a one in a million chance to survive the surgery."

The doctor turned to me. "Neil, if you want to tell them what you told me, go right ahead."

I said, "First, what choice do I have? And, as I told Dr. Domson when he said he had bad news, if I'm fortunate enough to come out the other side of this, God's going to have a plan for me, and if I don't come out on the other side, I won't know it."

In the face of this daunting diagnosis, something remarkable began to unfold. From the moment Darlene and I shared the news, my family and friends rallied around me with extraordinary and selfless acts of love and care. During the preparation for my critical surgery, through the grueling days of hospitalization, and throughout my challenging recovery at home, they were my lifeline. Their extraordinary and selfless acts—ranging from coordinating medical appointments to staying by my side in the hospital, from preparing meals to simply offering a comforting presence—became the bedrock of my strength. Through their incredible support, I found the courage to face each day, and their kindness illuminated the path to my recovery.

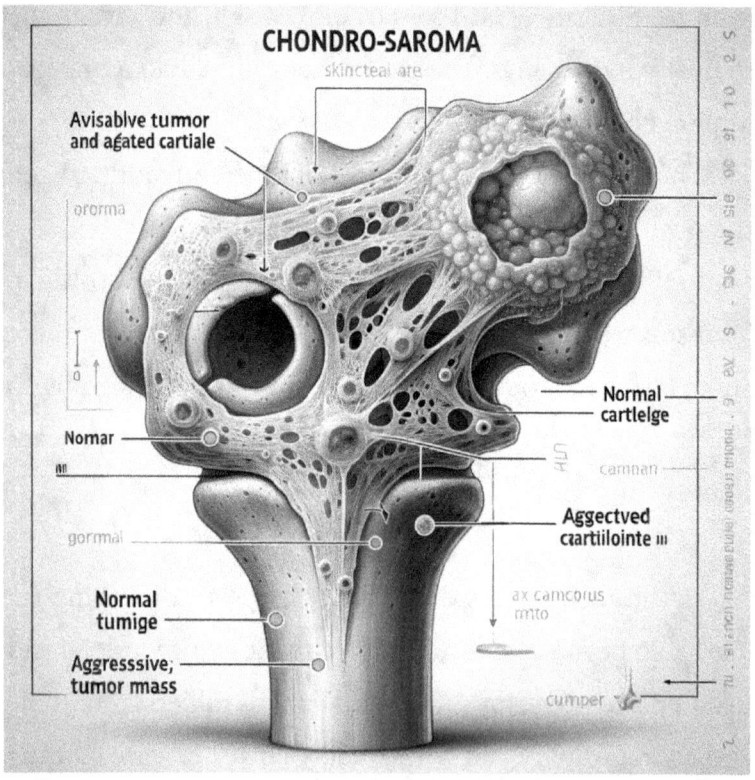

Chapter Three: Radiation Therapy

It wasn't long before the time came to return to Massachusetts General Hospital for six weeks of radiation therapy and I needed a place to stay. In my need to find an affordable place to stay during the six weeks of treatment, a friend who lives near Boston, Fred Tilley, pitched in to help. Fred is a colleague I'd worked with some years prior who at that time lived in Boston. An empty nester, he graciously offered to have me stay with him during that time. The hospital's concierge department, which had helped with our visit, offered access to area homes with families that had reasonable daily rates in comparison to hotels. My friend offered his home for free. The choice was simple and right—stay with my friend.

As I entered the Francis H. Burr Proton Therapy Center I wasn't the only one at Mass General for proton / photon radiation therapy. A lot of guys were having a proton beam aimed at their prostates, which is pretty common these days, but what I had is not exactly the same. The proton beam is pretty precise, and I had that, but I also had photon therapy, which goes all over the place. The proton beam goes exactly where they aim it. In my case, after the proton session, they would switch to photon therapy, which after attacking the marginal cells would

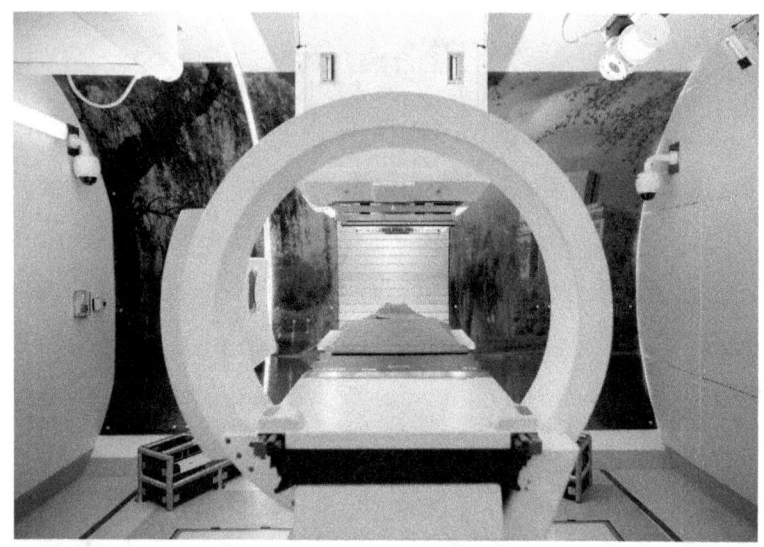

Proton Therapy Equipment

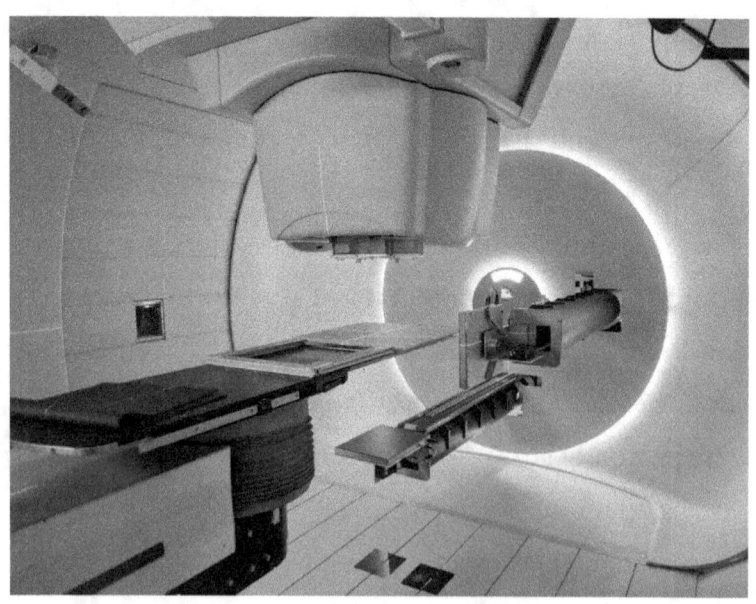

Self-Cured Addict

continue though my body and would scatter radiation particles all over the place. The people doing this would run to the inner depths of a lead-lined room before they turned on the photons because of how much those particles scatter—they bounce around for a long time. At the end, I'd lie there for about 20 minutes until the equipment indicated that the photons had cleared out of the air.

It takes quite an elaborate facility to house the proton beam and photon generator, which is basically an atomic accelerator. There are only two of them in the United States: The one at Mass General, consists of six linear accelerators located in the Lunder Building. Treatment planning for all proton-photon machines is performed using optimization techniques for the intense treatments. It's a massive commitment contained in a room eight floors beneath Boston.

I have to say, though, that six weeks of therapy was a great experience. Everyone there was amazed that I had no problems, no burning or blisters—no visible evidence of any kind that I'd had that type of therapy. Apparently, it was pretty unusual for a guy in his 60s—they were truly amazed. And something else—the therapy takes quite a while, and as you know, I had it every day for six weeks. To keep a patient from getting bored, they ask what kind of music you want to listen to. At first I said I didn't care—

Self-Cured Addict

that it didn't matter to me. Well, my son Devon was a popular private DJ at the time, and when he found out about it, he said I ought to liven things up a bit. He told me about some rappers whose songs ought to do the trick and suggested I let them know I wanted to listen to them. He gave me their names, and so I did. I'd go in and say I wanted to listen to current pop artisits. They would look at me, a guy in his 60s with whitening hair and start laughing. They were certainly surprised about my request but went ahead and played those songs. Devon had made a great suggestion because the staff looked forward to my visits from that day forward. While the radiation was going on, I could see them inside their control room laughing and groving to the music. I laughed with them. My impression was made. My approach to cancer would bring a fun experience to all.

Chapter Four: Prayer Works

Dr. Hornicek, whose wealth of knowledge and ability to relate everything through truth and kindness is invaluable, had authored numerous scholarly articles on the molecular biology of sarcomas, surgical techniques, and innovative treatments. At the time he was the department head and Professor at Harvard Medical School and the chief of the Musculoskeletal Oncology Service, the founder of the Stephen L. Harris Chordoma Center at Massachusetts General Hospital, and a professional with international recognition for his work in orthopedic oncology. I knew I had the best.

Dr. Hornicek at the time of this writing can be found as the Chair of the Department of Orthopedics, University of Miami Miller School of Medicine where he leads the department, focusing on expanding research initiatives and improving patient care within the orthopedic field. He told me up front, he didn't know if he'd be able to save my legs, but that he'd do his best. One likely had to go, but he said he'd do his best to save both of them. Regardless, however, one thing was certain. I would not be able to walk afterward.

In the operating room before that surgery, it was really cold—it seemed like it was about 50 degrees. A couple of dozen doctors and nurses were waiting to begin, and up above in a kind of balcony were another two dozen or so interns who were there to watch.

I told the anesthesiologist I wanted to have a minute of silence.

He nodded and said, "May I have your attention, everyone. Mr. Jackson has a special request. He'd like to have a moment of silence because he'd like to pray."

Then he looked at me and said, "It's all yours, Mr. Jackson."

I said, "I want a minute to pray, and you [those in the OR] to know, I'm not praying for me. I'm praying for you and you are welcome to join me in a moment of silence and prayer"

Then I said a prayer for them, and later I was told that it put everyone at ease.

Nevertheless, by the time I got done praying, I was crying like a baby.

The anesthesiologist said, "Are you done?"

I said, "Yes, I'm done. I'll count backwards."

He said, "Okay, let's get underway."

Frankly, I don't remember counting at all.

Let me say, parenthetically, that I prayed multiple times a day and before each surgery in the operating room, and that I deeply admire men and women who give prayer a high priority in their lives. Frankly, prayer has proved to be the most demanding discipline of my life. At different times, I have found it strenuous, boring, frustrating, and confusing. Over the years, maintaining a solid prayer life has been more intermittent than persistent. Admitting my lifelong struggle with prayer is something I do with great uneasiness.

From my experience, I have learned that you cannot simply "say your prayers." Prayer—real prayer—is tough, hard work. For me, prayer serves as preparation for battle, much like it did as I prepared for my surgery. I feel as though I have been on an incredible journey, a renewal of sorts, with God during the year leading up to my time at Mass General and throughout my stay there, that continues to this day. I believe this journey has been deeply influenced by what I've come to know as "The Brave Prayer," which I believe played a crucial role in my survival.

The Brave Prayer has become an essential aspect of my life, and I find it important to reflect on its significance. Lately, I've been contemplating just how impactful it must have been in my journey and my recovery. If you are not familiar with The Brave Prayer, I encourage you to look it up. It might just provide the strength and clarity you need in your own battles.

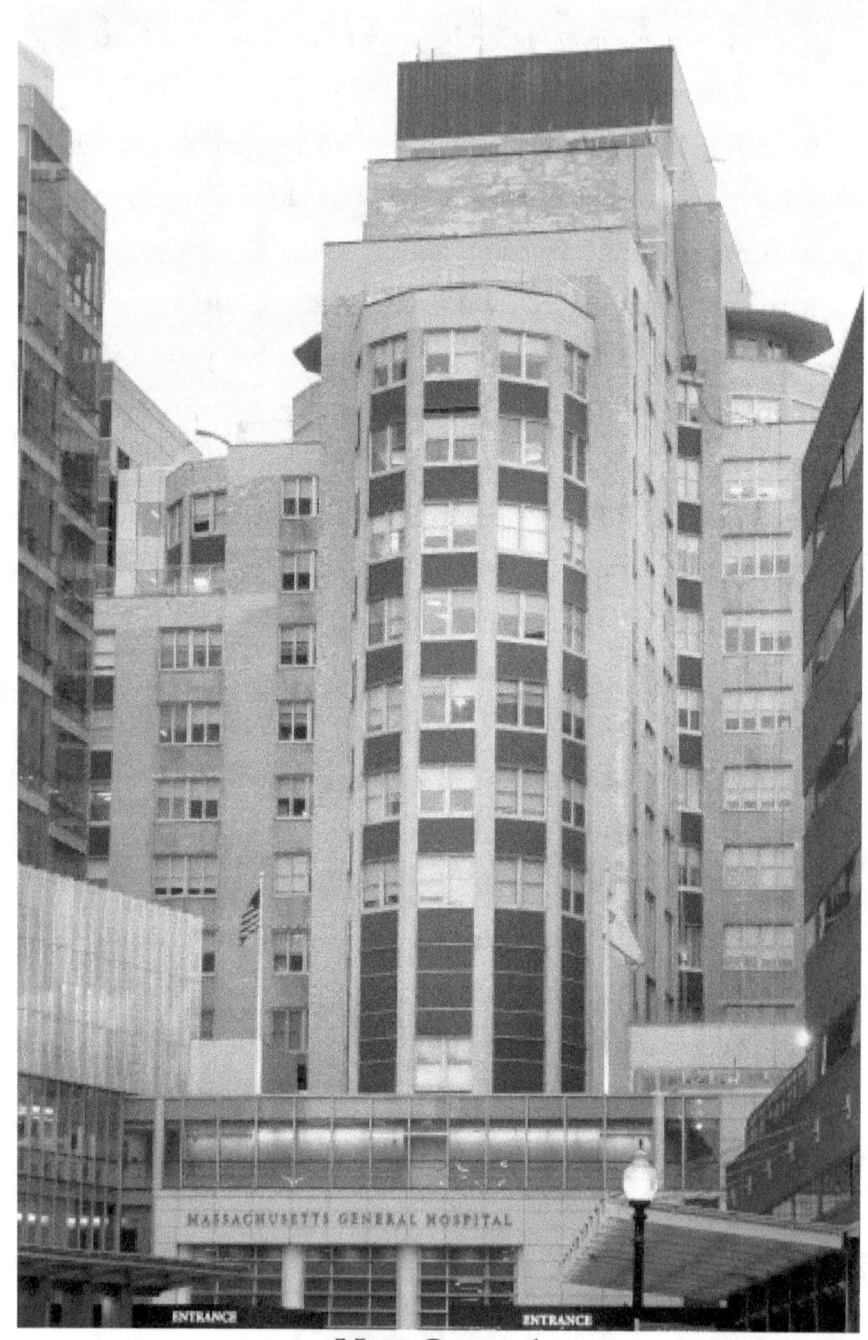

Mass General

Chapter Five: Surgery & the Aftermath

The surgery took twenty-one hours, over two sessions. The first, which had taken place a few days prior, was eight hours, the purpose of which was to prepare me for the second, which took thirteen hours. Because the tumor was wrapped around my pelvis and up my spine, I had to be positioned so that my head was down and my butt was up where they could work on it. The student's sight from above must have been sad!

According to Dr. Hornicek's surgical assisting doctor it was the first time he ever patted down his forehead from sweat in all previous surgeries. The surgery must have been an intense drama. At the conclusion Dr. Hornicek in full surgical garb walked into the waiting room and told Darlene, "You're not going to recognize your husband. His face is three times its normal size because of how we had to position him."

Miraculously, they were able to save both of my legs while I was to learn some devastating news about my spine later on.

I was in intensive care in a forced coma for more than a week. Once I came out of that and was moved to a normal room, in the cancer section immediately adjacent to the nursing station for the entire floor. I was given a morphine button that I could push whenever the pain got to be too much. The surgery had converted my aging body into a road map of incisions marked with hundreds of staples with protruding drainage and breathing tubes coming from all angles. Because I was bedridden with so many deep incisions, I was put on a special mattress that blows hot air and sand at about 85 degrees, which eliminated any breakdown of my skin. It was amazing. I was told the hospital rented this special bed for $550 a day—that was the hospital's cost. The result was that I had no skin breakdown at all even though I couldn't get out of bed for months.

The other not so good news was that my sacrum had been removed, which caused a serious problem. The sacrum is the triangular bone at the base of the spine and the center of the pelvis. It's made up of five fused vertebrae and forms the posterior wall of the pelvis. It connects the spine to the lower half of the body, stabilizes the pelvis, and helps control the bladder and bowels. The latter was the problem, the result of which was that I was always ringing a bell. I needed help because I'd crapped on myself, or whatever. All the healthcare providers at Mass General were kind and professional to the max, but nevertheless, I felt that my vanity was gone. I had no control at all.

Self-Cured Addict

A young and pretty night nurse came in one Friday and said, "I'm going to Vegas with my girlfriends, and I'll be back on Monday. I'd like a decision by then, and here's what I want you to decide about—a colostomy and a suprapubic tube." She tasked me to study the devices and decide whether to have the corrective procedures done. The next morning I began my studies.

A suprapubic tube goes into the bladder through your abdomen. A colostomy reroutes your colon through an opening that's made in the abdomen as well. Neither choice was pretty. In fact who would want these protrusions? Then again whoever invented them helps people like me live a normal life.

I called Darlene and explained the choice I'd been given, and I said, "I'm going to do it, I'm going to do both."

Darlene said, "Okay."

I said, "The reason I'm doing it is that you don't want me at home the way I am now. I would be an incredible burden. You couldn't work. I couldn't work. We'd be in a really bad place."

Then I called Dr. Hornicek's office, talked to Anne Fiore, his doctor of nurse practitioning, and told her what I was planning to do. She said she thought it was a great decision and that she'd tell Dr. Hornicek.

Dr. Hornicek called and said he thought it was a good decision and that he wanted to talk with me. So his office scheduled a medical transport [private ambulance] and I went to see him and told him I wanted both procedures done at the same time.

After the surgery I said to Darlene, "Now I can travel from Lynchburg to Miami, and I don't have to get out of the car for anything." There was still a lot of healing to take place before that could occur.

All in all, I was in the hospital for seven weeks prior to the surgery to have the proton beam and photon therapy and for eleven months that included surgeries and for recuperation after the surgery. The total cost was $2.2 million, which was paid by Lynchburg's privately owned regional Piedmont Health System Insurance with the support of our family physician, Dr. Smith, a kind and generous professional. But not everything was covered. The big thing was transportation costs. The Spaulding Rehabilitation Center, where I went after about five months to spend the rest of the eleven months, was about a mile from the hospital. Whenever I needed to see the doctor or some test was needed, an ambulance would be sent to get me. The cost of that was $1400 each way. Over the course of that time, we accumulated an outstanding bill with Mass General including other charges totaling $88,000. The pressure to pay intensified daily and began to tear at the fabric of my family. As a result, we ended up having to declare bankruptcy where the hospital received about ten cents on the dollar outstanding. If there is a need to address the overpricing of health care maybe start with the supporting services sector like transportation. The transportation fee systems appear to be huge profit centers that warrant review.

Chapter Six: Back Home in Lynchburg

Let me tell you about the trip home from Boston to Lynchburg. A good friend I've now known for about 50 years helped out. His name is John Moore, and he was my boss at Central Fidelity. John came to the bank from KPMG, the accounting firm, to be the audit director, and we worked together from the mid 1970s until the bank was purchased in 1998. About ten years after that, around 2008, we started working together again as consultants to various businesses.

John was a great friend. Both Darlene and I talked with him frequently from right after the diagnosis all the way through the time that I was finally discharged from MGH. It's great to have someone with whom you can share concerns—someone who listens, understands and offers comfort and support. We continue to keep in touch today on a regular basis.

When the time came for me to come home after almost a year in Boston, John, who then lived in Richmond, drove to Lynchburg and accompanied Darlene from Lynchburg to Boston on the train. They took the train because I'd left my car at the friend's house where I'd stayed

Self-Cured Addict

while having radiation therapy. Anyhow, John and Darlene went and got my car, and then they came and got me at the rehabilitation center. Darlene sat in the front seat, John drove, and I had the entire backseat to myself.

It was a long trip, and of course we had to stop for gas and to eat, but we wanted to get home as soon as possible, and so we did not take any side trips or spend any more time than necessary off the road. Typically, we'd pull off at a rest stop on whatever turnpike we happened to be on. We did, however, spend one night on the way with a friend in Jersey. As I recall, because of my wheelchair, we had some trouble getting in and out of his house.

Once back in Lynchburg I had to undergo physical rehab. I was placed on a bed that didn't have a floating sheet, and within days my skin broke down. Treatment was provided by the wound center. However after being released from rehab and within a brief period of time the skin breakdown got so infected that the metal inside my hip was visible. It smelled horrible and was truly a mess. It was evident that the hospital's wound center did not know how to stop the infection and remained silent about the growing danger. We took pictures of it and sent them to Dr. Hornicek.

He called right away and said, "Get up here as fast as possible."

When I arrived, after assessing the infection the doctors said stopping the numerous staff infections that existed would take time. It took three weeks before surgery could be done. I had to take five antibiotics through a shunt directly into my heart. During those weeks, I would be taken directly into the operating room where a power washer was used to clean out the infection. The surgeons who worked on me said they had never seen a situation so bad. Frankly, and truthfully, it stank.

Dr. Hornicek was extremely angry about it. He said, "If you want to sue those people in Lynchburg, we'll come to testify on your behalf at our own expense."

I understood why he felt that way. He and the Mass General doctors [all chiefs of their departments] had worked in and out of the operating room with MIT and Harvard Medical School, using imaging services to design and create different replacement pelvises and hips to select from and use during the original surgery, and now all of that was for naught.

Because there was infected flesh around metal, and antibiotics do not cure infections in flesh that's around metal, if they could save the leg I would need a shunt into my hip for the rest of my life, feeding the wound antibiotics. I said I didn't want a box on my abdomen or somewhere around there that had to be refilled all the time and

Self-Cured Addict

was told the alternative was to remove my leg, which would be major surgery. There was a chance I would die, because one of the major arteries—the femoral artery—had to be cut.

Dr. Hornicek and Dr. Schwab, who would perform the surgery explained all that and gave me the choice.

So I said, "Just take the leg off. I don't have a choice, let's get it done. You're the best in the world. If you can't do it, no one can. If it doesn't work out, my family will not have any problems with it."

As mentioned earlier, I found that when you say something like that to a doctor, especially those doctors, it takes the pressure off and puts them at ease.

To conclude the story about the infection, I decided that while suing was an option, it would only destroy the doctor. Although I believe he did make mistakes, he was not someone I wanted to destroy. It was nearing Christmas so I emailed Dr. Hornicek and told him my decision and wished him a Merry Christmas as I awaited the removal of my leg. If it had been the hospital alone, my decision to sue would have been different. I learned the power of forgiveness and continue to benefit from it today.

Chapter Seven: The Wake Up Call

Perhaps it's surprising, but I didn't think of myself as being addicted to opioids, nor did I consider what I quickly realized was the need to hoard drugs to be anything other than reflective of my professional background, which involved risk mitigation, reducing the possibility of being without pain medication. The way I thought went something like this: Suppose it snows today, and we can't get to the pharmacy? Suppose it's time to renew my prescription and my doctor says "no?" In order to protect myself, I believed I needed to put drugs aside. I had to figure out a way to do that, and so I had a conversation with my pharmacist.

I said, "When can I get these renewals done?"

He said, "The insurance company will authorize payment three days before the renewal day as long as the prescriptions are on file."

So I would call over to my doctor's office, and say I needed a renewal. They would send it over to Walmart pharmacy, and I would go and get it three days early.

Imagine getting prescriptions three days early over a period of seven years. During that time you are going to accumulate a lot of extra pills, and that's what I did. It seems crazy, but I was taking six hydromorphone pills a day, six oxycontin pills, and maybe six gabapentin pills a day. So all those pills started to accumulate. At the same time, I was experiencing some fluctuations in pain and I needed to get that straightened out.

I knew a pharmacist who had been a neighbor of mine when we owned our house, and he agreed to help manage my medication and to get it straightened out. He had observed me all over the place—drugged up, vomiting, and with splitting headaches, chronic pain and depression. Something needed to be done. So working with my personal physician we quickly exchanged and seriously lowered the dosage quantity of hydrocodone pills by offsetting them with hydromorphone pills and a transdermal fentanyl patch. What the doctor and the pharmacist decided was that the even flow of the drug administered by the transdermal patch without going through my digestive tract would produce a more even and non-disruptive state of relief. Also, there would be no more oral intake than necessary to service spikes in pain if this occurred. Gabapentin which was a part of the store of drugs didn't bother my digestive system and hydromorphone didn't, but oxycontin and hydrocodone were giving me a lot of problems. So we replaced them and things stabilized as a result while dependency quietly grew.

Nevertheless, two weeks after I started morphine and got into hydrocodone, hydromorphone and gabapentin at the hospital, like others, I was addicted—some may call it dependent, but I didn't know it. All I knew back then was that I needed to push the button and take the pills because I was in severe chronic pain, and those pills killed the pain, and when the pain returned, I knew it.

When I was in the hospital, and the pain came, I would hit the morphine button or call the nurse on duty to give me something additional to relieve extreme pain. Sometimes a nurse would come into my room and say the doctor would have to approve it.

I'd say, "Hell, you know me, I've been here for months and this [need for relief] happens all the time."

The doctors at Mass General knew me, and yet they were still hesitant to give me drugs at the exact time that I wanted them. They had to approve the request, and once they did, I got them, but it would sometimes take an hour or two. Then the transition into treating the pain took hours as well. It was hell at times.

So once I was at home in Lynchburg, I didn't want to end my use of drugs, and go to an independent drug rehabilitative services center because I realized that if I was in a rehab center, they wouldn't know me or care about me. If I went to rehab services, I'd have to give them all my drugs when I came in, and I wasn't about to give in knowing I needed drugs, I was afraid of the pain. I figured at the very least I was going to get into an argument if I asked for drugs, and I didn't want that. So I immediately rejected the idea of going to Drug Rehabilitative Services.

My next option was what's called Medicated Alternate Treatment (MAT) where doctors would likely use Suboxone in an effort to transition me off the drugs I was on. Suboxone is a combination of two drugs, Buprenorphine and Naloxone. Apparently, Buprenorphine binds to and partially activates opioid receptors, which decreases opioid withdrawal symptoms. But I'd read enough about these things to know that Suboxone is an addictive drug. It is presented as not quite as extreme as fentanyl or Hydromorphone, in the dependency / addiction concern which both are [FDA] Schedule Two narcotics. Instead, as a [FDA] Schedule One drug I learned that it teeters on Schedule Two classification, which means there actually isn't a great deal of difference. I also learned that ending the use of Suboxone is actually more difficult than fentanyl or other opioids including heroin. So now knowing that I figured I'd just be trading the drug dependency I already had for a new one, which did not make a lot of sense to me. So I told myself what I needed to do was to find another way, and eventually, that's what I did. A strong impetus to do so came on November 1, 2017.

It seems to me that some things are meant to be—what the famous psychiatrist Carl Jung called, "synchronicities," which as mentioned in Chapter One are meaningful coincidences that on the surface seem to have no obvious or logical cause. One happened to me when I was watching the news on television one morning. I had reached the end of a program, and switched to C-SPAN to see if anything interesting was going on. Well, it was. President Trump was in the Rose Garden with several officials from his administration and a gaggle of reporters. I decided to watch because at that time President Trump was still something of a novelty to me, and so I decided to see what was going on in the White House. Lo and behold, former New Jersey Governor, Chris Christie, then Chairman of the Opioid and Drug Abuse Commission was giving a report on a study that President Trump had assigned him to lead concerning the epidemic of opioid and drug abuse that was going on across the country. In that Rose Garden ceremony on November 1, 2017, President Trump declared the opioid crisis a public health emergency and released, "The Commission's Report on Combating Drug Addiction and the Opioid Crisis."

> "If you have a dirty fish tank, you clean it. You do not drug the fish." —unknown source

As you can imagine, I listened and later read the report intently, and in doing so my eyes were opened wide to the

Self-Cured Addict

hazards and ills these drugs brought with them. For example, I learned that fentanyl and other opioids kill brain cells—that it had been found from the examination of individuals who'd died from addiction and drug overdoses that the matter that surrounded their brains had turned from gray to white. When I heard about this and other findings, I was quite frankly shocked. So I went online and downloaded the full report.

When I read what they had been talking about, I picked up the phone, called Darlene, told her about it and added, "Those b****ds were talking to me." In other words, I had accepted what they said fully—all of it, hook, line, and sinker. I also said I was certain there was a reason I had turned on C-SPAN that morning. It was not something I often did. Was this another pathway presented by God to unfold my new mission I had earlier stated to Dr. Domson that would come in my "coming out the other side of surgery?"

The bottom line in my mind was that I had to do something as soon as possible. As I read through the report, I decided to Google some of the medical terms that had been used, and the images that came up were awfully scary. For example, the image of a normal brain came up that was juxtaposed with one that had been ravaged by drugs. The matter around the affected brain was turning white and disappearing—a person with a brain like that would soon be dead.

I began to wonder where my brain might be on the continuum, and hoped to God I was still at a point where I could recover. I figured I needed to get off the drugs I was taking as quickly as possible. The only question was, "How?"

As mentioned above I never thought I was addicted. The word, "addicted" didn't enter my mind until Darlene and I went up to the University of Virginia Medical Center, and we met with the pain management director for the hospital.

For some reason the realization I was addicted came to me, and I said to her, "Damn, I'm addicted to these drugs."

She said, "You're not addicted."

I said, "What am I?"

She said, "You're dependent."

I said, "What's the difference?"

This angered me so much that I told Darlene, "We're out of here."

Anyhow, I found out what I needed to know on that trip—I had a serious problem. So I began to research the options.

Self-Cured Addict

How I Became Free of Hydromorphone

I was determined to free myself from the grip of opioids, and it seemed to me the place to start was with Hydromorphone. Commonly known by the brand name Dilaudid, Hydromorphone is a potent opioid pain medication that I was taking in pill form.

The initial phase of my tapering process commenced on April 8, 2018. That's when I opted to tackle what at the time seemed to be the simplest aspect of my addiction. Using a modified pill cutter, I began the meticulous task of slicing the hydromorphone pills. This methodical "slicing process" required precision to ensure that each pill was chipped, sliced, or shaved into uniform particles over the course of the next six months, gradually reducing them from full four-milligram pills to minuscule addiction-ending fragments.

At the outset, my prescribed dosage of hydromorphone (Dilaudid) consisted of eight milligrams every six hours. I initiated the slicing regimen on a bi-weekly basis, adjusting the frequency of tapering based on what I felt to be the impact of each reduction. As time progressed, I found myself increasing the frequency to a weekly basis, ultimately concluding the process on August 6, 2018. While my method may have seemed rudimentary, it worked. Through slow, deliberate chipping away, I meticulously documented any physical changes, and surprisingly, there were none. I also made note of my mental and attitudinal shifts, which I can only categorize as positive. Some days, I noticed subtle shifts in mood, while others marked the absence of debilitating migraine headaches, persistent nausea and times of deep depression.

Overall, my notes revealed a remarkable absence of the anticipated pain which I feared most "residual pain" stemming from my cancer surgery. Reflecting on this journey, I couldn't help but wonder why I hadn't embarked on this path to freedom from addiction years earlier.

Having successfully tapered off hydromorphone, my next challenge was to discontinue the use of fentanyl, a significantly more potent and addictive opioid, a task that presented daunting hurdles.

I Invent a Way to Free Myself from Fentanyl

Eventually, I came up with the idea to block in a graduated and managed way the transdermal flow of fentanyl from the patch to my skin, starting with a small non-permeable barrier, and slowly increasing the size of the barrier and amount of blockage over time until no fentanyl got through and I was free of the drug. The question was how. What could I use to block the flow?

The first thing I tried was artists' tape. You see, I'm an artist who uses thin artists' tape to create fine lines. So I

Self-Cured Addict

took some of my tape to see if it would block the flow of the drug from the patch to my skin. I figured it wouldn't kill me to partially block the flow because I could easily pull off the tape and return to the flow of fentanyl to normal if I needed to. So I tried it, and it didn't do a thing—the fentanyl ate right through the tape. It simply didn't block it. I could see fentanyl on the other side next to my skin. Obviously, I had to find a material that fentanyl didn't and couldn't penetrate, and so I started to search and to experiment until I did finally find one material that worked to block the drug.

I started by using that material to cover what I calculated to be five percent of the patch. Going forward, I would cut the barrier material into strips that would reduce the flow of the drug from the patch to my skin by certain percentages that would grow according to what coverage size I calculated. When I started, I was receiving 100 micrograms per hour every 48 hours in contrast to the normal prescribed 72 hour use of patches. This was in response to my growing demand and is a really high dosage. From there, I decreased the flow at a slow and steady pace with my physician as my coach over a 14 month period until I was completely free of the drug.

You may wonder if I was in any pain or other discomforts after I was free of fentanyl. I had read that nerves regenerate about one inch a year, and that once the regeneration starts, the nerve endings are healing themselves. I figured if I had residual pain, I could always go back to taking the drugs, but I did not have any residual pain—at least not from the surgery to remove the tumor. I did, however, have phantom pain because of the amputation of my leg, which apparently is common with amputees. My other challenges of nausea, migraines, depression and low blood pressure were gone or seriously reduced to what we could consider normal. The phantom pain, not relieved by opioids, comes and goes mainly based on the weather, and I deal with it when needed using either Motrin and Tylenol—neither of which are addictive.

Another synchronicity occurred when I was almost completely free of fentanyl and visiting my friend, Jim Parker.

Jim is a retired electrical engineer who happens to have thirty or so patents on devices he created. We were in his garage, and I was telling him how I'd been able to wean myself off the drug.

His interest perked, and he said, "Show me what you've been doing."

I opened my shirt and showed him the patch.

He said, "That's it? That's what you call 'your barrier'?"

"Right."

Self-Cured Addict

He said, "You do know, don't you—that's patentable?"

Well, that blew my mind. Over the years, I'd launched a number of businesses and enterprises with some success and with some not so successful. It was a passion of mine, and so the minute I got back to my apartment that day, I drafted an email to Dr. Francis Collins, then the head of the National Institutes of Health, in order to find out if Jim Parker was right. Along with it, I also sent Dr. Collins a description of the product, which I think was fairly well written if I do say so myself.

Dr. Collins called me right away and said that what I had was the solution to a national epidemic—that he'd never seen anything like it from a patient before. He went on to say he was going to put me together with his deputy at the National Institute of Drug Abuse, and that he would instruct his deputy to help guide me through the process in order to get the product into the marketplace as quickly as possible.

From that point, we were off to the races. We teamed up with Dr. Gerry Moeller, a Professor and Division Chair for Addiction Psychiatry in the Department of Addiction Psychiatry, and Dr. Matthew Halquist, Associate Professor and Director, Bioanalytical Shared Resource Laboratory at the Virginia Commonwealth University Medical Center. Working with them, we prepared to apply to NIDA for grant funding in the amount of $3.5 million, which is what Dr. Moeller estimated with the consultation of NIDA would be required to fund the necessary research.

It looked like we were going to get it submitted when the COVID-19 pandemic came along, and tragically, the National Institutes of Health stopped all funding for research except that which had to do with COVID.

When that happened, I talked with Dr. Moeller at VCU Medical. He said he had no idea what the timeline was or would be. As a medical research facility, VCU Medical was hurting overall because of the action by NIH. Grants were hugely important to them.

With all the uncertainty, I decided not to wait. I told him I was going to try to get things going privately.

Dr. Moeller said, "That's a huge task, Neil."

He was right. As of this writing, it has been four years since COVID began, and only recently has the FenBlock device begun its submission into the FDA for clearance.

Rest assured, however, that we are doing all we can to get FenBlock approved and into the hands of doctors. Meanwhile, the epidemic of drug abuse and the deaths caused by it continue to plague our country and much of the world.

Chapter Eight: The Cure

Upon approval by the FDA, FenBlock's patented barrier technology will present a promising solution for individuals looking to reduce their dependence on Schedule Two narcotics, including both prescribed controlled substances and illicit opioids such as fentanyl. Here's a comprehensive overview of how FenBlock's innovative approach works:

Initial Assessment and Customized Plan

The process should begin with an initial assessment by a physician to understand the patient's current use, dependency level, and overall health. Based on this thorough evaluation, a customized reduction plan should be developed to meet the specific needs and circumstances of the individual.

How FenBlock's Barrier Technology Works

FenBlock employs a patented novel barrier technology designed with the oversight of a physician to:

- **Gradually Reduce Absorption**: This technology minimizes the absorption of the narcotic into the bloodstream, thereby lessening its overall effect.

- **Mitigate Withdrawal Symptoms**: By gradually decreasing the body's dependency on the narcotic, FenBlock helps to ease withdrawal symptoms.
- **Gradual and Managed Dependency Reduction**: The technology supports a step-by-step reduction in narcotic use, allowing the body to adjust slowly and comfortably.

Ongoing Monitoring and Support

Regular check-ups with the physician are recommended and are an integral part of the process. These visits ensure:

- **Progress Monitoring**: Physicians can track the patient's progress and make necessary adjustments to the reduction plan.
- **Comprehensive Support**: Additional resources such as counseling, support groups, and other services should be made available to address the psychological and social aspects of dependency.

Combining Technology with Medical Oversight

FenBlock's approach is highly effective because it integrates advanced risk free medical device technology with continuous medical oversight and robust private or publicly available support systems. This combination creates a structured and supportive environment that promotes healthier, drug-free lives by empowering the patient through personal accomplishments and significantly reduces recidivism.

Getting More Information

For more detailed information on FenBlock's barrier technology and its applications, please visit FenBlock's official website by scanning the QR code below or consult with a medical professional who is familiar with this innovative approach.

By leveraging FenBlock's barrier technology under the guidance of healthcare professionals, individuals struggling with dependency on Schedule Two narcotics can find a safe path to recovery that is both manageable and sustainable.

Postscript

Emotions can dramatically and without judgment alter the course of recovery as I learned on a fateful morning in December 2012 during the best times of my recovery and rehabilitation. I had returned to MGH with a serious set of infections and was awaiting surgery that eventually would take my left leg. The air in the hospital room was thick with the sterile scent of antiseptic and the quiet hum of medical machinery. I lay in my bed, confined to limited movement, feeling the weight of my 63 years and the burden, or was it the reward of my recent cancer surgery. The doctors had called it a miracle—a one in a million chance of surviving such a complicated, incurable cancer. I was still grappling with the gravity of my situation when the headlines of the *Boston Herald* arrived, forever altering my emotional landscape.

The pathology report that had come back during my earlier stay and after the cancer surgery was clearly to the absolute pleasure of the surgeons, nurses and, of course, my family. It could have been, "we were unable to get it all, and we expect the cancer to return with a vengeance and quickly." Death could have been around the corner. Why had I been marked for survival? By whom and why? This question came to my mind in the early morning while

Self-Cured Addict

watching TV. The date was December 14, 2012, and the headline of a NEWSBREAK on the local Boston morning news program screamed tragedy: a gunman had entered Sandy Hook Elementary School in Newtown, Connecticut, and taken the lives of 26 innocent souls, including 20 young children.

As I learned the details, tears welled up in my eyes, and a deep, uncontrollable sobbing overtook me. The overwhelming grief and horror of the event clashed violently with the relief and gratitude I was supposed to feel about my own survival.

Why had I been spared when so many innocent children had not? This question haunted me, casting a dark shadow over my upcoming surgery and recovery. I felt an intense, almost suffocating conflict in my heart and mind. It seemed incomprehensible that a loving God could permit such a heinous act to occur while allowing me, a person in the twilight of life battling an incurable disease, to continue living. The contrast was unbearable, and the guilt of surviving gnawed at my spirit.

In those initial days of recovery, my mind was a battlefield. I recalled a conversation with my oncologist where I spoke of a sense of mission and purpose. Could this survival be part of a predetermined plan? Was there a reason I was still here, a mission I was meant to fulfill? The search for answers seemed futile, the pain of the children's loss too raw and immediate.

Each night, I would cry myself to sleep, grappling with the notion of divine will and the randomness of life. The headlines kept replaying in my mind, each child's face a poignant reminder of life's fragility and my own fortunate escape. Should I deny my survival, view it as an undeserved gift, and feel guilty for living while they perished? Or should I seek deeper meaning, find or create an answer to this existential dilemma?

The answer, I found, lay in a childhood lesson that had been my beacon through many storms: prayer. In prayer, I sought solace and understanding. I was an emotional wreck, likely due to the incredible dosages of opioids flooding my body. In the absence of answers, I turned to prayer. Through prayer, I expressed my anguish, confusion, trust, hope, and gratitude. Slowly, I began to accept that some questions may never have clear answers, that faith often means trusting without understanding.

Prayer became my refuge, a way to reconcile the paradox of my survival and their loss. It allowed me to leave my doubts and fears at the feet of the Lord, trusting that He had a plan far beyond my comprehension. This acceptance did not erase the pain or the questions, but it gave me a framework within which to place them.

As I wrote this book and told my story, the impact of that tragic event remained profound. It has reshaped my understanding of life and survival, imbuing it with a sense of responsibility and purpose. My journey through this emotional conflict has strengthened my faith, teaching me to lean on prayer and to trust in the Lord's wisdom, even when faced with the inexplicable.

Reflections

The journey through such personal and emotional conflict is deeply transformative. It teaches that positive emotions bound by personal faith and convictions centered on survival, especially against insurmountable odds, can carry a profound sense of purpose and reinforce the values and strength found in Christ through prayer. I believe that strength and sense of purpose is available to others who seek it, which underscores the importance I place in my faith and prayers in their ability to help me navigate life, even in its darkest moments. Throughout this story, I hope I have conveyed the resilience of the human spirit and the healing power of faith.

In the face of tragedy or difficult challenges, and in survival, finding peace is such an important process. It involves embracing the unknown, seeking solace through Christ, and allowing prayer to guide the heart towards acceptance. This story is meant to be a testament to the enduring strength found in spiritual faith and the quest for meaning in the aftermath of unimaginable events.

PART TWO
Thoughts, Reflections,
& Recommendations

Author's Note

Anyone who has successfully traversed the twelve step program prescribed by Alcoholics Anonymous will tell you that belief and faith in a higher power is essential to overcoming an addiction, and I found that to be true as well. In fact, as a devout Christian, I experienced an unexpected and profound sense of peace in the midst of turmoil. The same is true for any religion where we acknowledge a power greater than ourselves. In a moment of clarity, I felt compelled to embrace my oncologist's diagnosis as a divine gift, a pivotal turning point orchestrated by God Himself. With unwavering faith, I expressed to my physician, "I believe this is a gift from God, and it will ultimately be for the best. If I am fortunate enough to emerge from the surgery victorious, God will reveal His plan for me." In that moment, I understood the importance of surrendering to God's will and placing my trust entirely in His divine guidance.

Under the expert care of Dr. Francis Hornicek and Dr. Joseph Schwab at Massachusetts General Hospital (MGH), and a host of other chiefs of departments and full professors at Harvard Medical School, they shared valuable insights acquired from their extensive chondrosacroma experience, noting the rarity of encountering "class two" and "class three" cancer cells without the presence of more advanced stages such as "class four" cells, the most aggressive.

As you know, he also spoke candidly about my chances for survival. With my wife Darlene at my side and in front of the chiefs and senior assisting specialists in the meeting who would participate in the procedures he stated that in his opinion I faced a one in one million chance of surviving surgery.

Something I did not mention in Part One is that seven months after the surgery and prior to my release from MGH Dr. Hornicek modified his predictive number from one million to three million due to the complexities that occurred within the many hours of surgery that took place.

Guided by the teachings encapsulated in the Bible and the book *Crossing the Threshold of Hope*, authored by His Holiness, Pope John Paul II, I found guidance, solace, and inspiration. Embracing the timeless wisdom encapsulated in the teaching of John 6:20, "It is I; do not be afraid," that many times is worded "Be Not Afraid," drawn from the words of Jesus and His disciples, I discovered a source of unwavering courage. This newfound perspective imbued me with a profound sense of acceptance and confidence, propelling me forward to confront the trials of surgery and treatment with steadfast determination. The book never left my bedside. It's still on my desk as I write today.

Self-Cured Addict

The inadequacies of my misconceptions were revealed by my visual encounter.

Little did I realize the profound impact of my acceptance and the transformative journey that lay ahead, not only for myself but also for my family. Upon receiving the sobering news of my diagnosis, a friend extended an invitation for lunch and gave me a book titled *In a Pit with a Lion on a Snowy Day*, by Mark Batterson, the Lead Pastor at National Community Church in Washington, DC. This literary treasure served as a wellspring of inspiration, further infusing me with the energy needed to confront the impending challenges of my surgery. Carrying the Bible and both books and the teachings encapsulated within each I found solace and strength within their pages, recommending them all wholeheartedly to anyone grappling with life's formidable trials. The last pathway in my increasing faith before entering the hospital for surgery was a printed paper a motel manager gave me upon learning I was at MGH for cancer. I had crossed through the lobby heading for the restaurant out front when she said hello. When I replied she undoubtedly recognized a Virginia accent and asked where I was from. That lead to her telling me about the power of St. Peregrine, the Catholic Patron Saint of Cancer. She told me to recite the Peregrin Pray three times a day and I would be fine. I did and I am. No further explanation needed.

Have you ever felt like you were stumbling around in the dark, unsure of your path or purpose? That was where I was before everything changed when I received that life-altering diagnosis. You may be as I was before that fateful day—shadowed by doubt or discouragement. But I want to remind you that you, as I, were never meant to live in darkness.

When we allow His light to illuminate our lives, something beautiful happens. We begin to see ourselves as He sees us—beloved, valuable, and filled with potential. We discover a purpose that transcends our circumstances, a joy that outweighs our sorrows, and a hope that anchors us in the storms of life. My mission became clear: helping others end their use of fentanyl and opioids. This mission, which took seven years to develop, has become my life's work.

Today, I encourage you to seek and embrace your God-given call to shine. Be patient in His direction. As you find your mission, step out of the shadows of fear and insecurity, and trust that the glory of the Lord is risen upon you. You were created to be a light, and the world needs the unique glow that only you can bring.

Self-Cured Addict

Shining is not just in some of us; it's in everyone. We are all meant to shine. As we let our own light shine, we give others permission to do the same. As we are liberated from our own fears, our presence automatically liberates others.

> "Arise, shine, for your light has come, and the glory of the Lord rises upon you." – Isaiah 60:1

Embrace your light and let it shine brightly, for this is our time to illuminate the world with hope, love, and purpose.

Future Hope

"The time has come," he said. "The kingdom of God has come near. Repent and believe the good news." —Mark 1:15

Introduction to Part Two

In recent years, the scourge of opioids and narcotics has escalated into a widespread epidemic, posing formidable challenges to society and government, not only in the United States but around the globe. The roots of addiction often trace back to gateway drugs like marijuana, which can and do serve as precursors to more potent substances. The proliferation of prescribed fentanyl and other opioid pain medication has only exacerbated the crisis, serving as feeder drugs that fuel the cycle of addiction that leads many, which nearly included me, to street solutions and possible death. These substances, originally intended for legitimate medical use, have been exploited and abused, leading many down the perilous, unforgiving path of dependency, addiction, and despair. The expanding reach of prescribed fentanyl and opioids, underscores the need for comprehensive prescription and insurance payer reform, support of innovation in treatment, and oversight of intervention efforts by physicians and medical providers to combat this devastating challenge and offer hope to those ensnared in its grasp. Combining the destiny of a chronic pain patient for life with the escalating challenges and epidemic of prescribed as well as illicit opioid use, abuse, dependency and addiction, I found myself surrounded by personal and societal problems I never anticipated I would have to address.

Not long after being prescribed opioids, I found myself using fentanyl for pain relief only to be ensnared in the insidious grasp of addiction to the highest allowed daily dosage of fentanyl and other opioids. What initially served as a beacon of relief from my chronic pain soon morphed into a relentless battle against dependency and addiction. With each passing day, I felt the suffocating weight of growing dependency tightening its grip, rendering me captive to its chains demanding increased prescriptions from my physicians.

Yet, I was determined not to succumb to despair. Fueled by an unyielding faith and resolve and an unwavering determination to reclaim my freedom and health, I embarked on a journey of self-discovery and innovation. Drawing upon my own harrowing experiences and the invaluable insights gained from the arduous struggle, I set forth to forge a solution—a beacon of hope for myself and what has turned out to be that for countless others ensnared in a similar plight.

It was not too late. Fueled by a burning and impassioned new purpose in life and desire to effect positive change, I poured my heart and soul and entire retirement funds into the creation of FenBlock—a patented, graduated, and scalable tapering medical device meticulously designed to

Self-Cured Addict

offer respite to those dependent and addicted to fentanyl patches. My justification remains, it is not about me that I came across FenBlock. Rather it is about you, that is now my mission. Dr. Francis Collins termed it "the first patient driven solution to a national epidemic." Day and night for more than four years, I labored tirelessly in my makeshift laboratory, fueled solely by sheer determination and an unwavering faith and a stellar mission founded in a new purpose in life.

With each iteration of FenBlock crafted and each obstacle overcome, I inched closer to realizing my vision of a world where fentanyl addiction, prescribed and illicit, need no longer be synonymous with despair and destruction. After months of relentless dedication and countless setbacks and two steps forward, I proudly unveiled FenBlock to the world. My invention was met with reverence and acclaim—a beacon of hope illuminating the path to recovery for millions ensnared in the clutches of fentanyl addiction. As I write these words, my invention is with the FDA which hopefully will expedite its approval.

Through FenBlock, I not only vanquished my own demons but also I believe I have paved the way for countless others to reclaim freedom, their lives, and to rewrite their destinies. Armed with my invention and an unyielding determination to effect change. I hope and pray that the story told in Part One of this book emerges as a beacon of hope and inspiration for others—a testament to the transformative power of God, personal resilience, innovation, and the indomitable human spirit.

"What is it [addiction]?" We need to know before we call ourselves addicted. We are not alone in our possible confusion over our status, which may lie somewhere between user, dependent user, or addictive user. Who decides and under what [standard] measurements? Psychiatrists, psychologists, chemical dependency counselors, and people like you and me the world over beginning, or in recovery programs, are constantly asking this question. Neuroscientists have entered the fray, searching for both the cause and effective management of addiction. Yet there is no consensus. Defining addiction remains an area of heated debate. Yet despite differences of opinion, most of us can recognize—and through recognition, perhaps better understand—certain behaviors and situations in which "normal" use of addictive drugs turns to destructive dependency. I did and I found myself in heated debate concerning how to safely end my addiction and use with minimal impact in the form of withdrawal.

Self-Cured Addict

Most people who become addicted become enchained to their drug of choice (illicit) or to the drug chosen for them (prescribed). The word "addiction" comes from the Latin verb "addicere," which means to give over, dedicate or surrender. For many reasons, some people begin to wriggle against the chains of addiction. Whether it is because they have experiences that scare them to death (not uncommon and exactly my experience) or lose something that really matters (also not uncommon), some people begin to work themselves out of the chains. People whose descent into addiction came later in life have more memories of what life can be like free of their use of and addiction to drugs. Some like me have been blessed and will be able to turn and see the fire. Those who started so young that it is all they really know often experience fear and confusion. But as sometimes happens in recovery, they can start to come out of the cave of darkness as well.

There is a growing misunderstanding of what constitutes fentanyl and other opioid addiction. Discussions throughout communities today focus heavily on illicit fentanyl and fentanyl laced drugs that are wreaking havoc on society. Is addiction without reason? Does it seem to involve a total abdication of reason? Is it just a messy tangle of emotions and a lack of will? I say these are interesting questions that a therapist may address, but they are not the essence of who we are—those of us who desire to return to normal health and end their addiction and use of fentanyl and other opioids.

As an addict whose pathway began with prescribed opioid pain medication I came very close to entering street and illicit drugs. My path represents an under-discussed feeder path that leads from prescribed to illicit narcotics. My path is symbolic of many others who, unlike me, took the step to enter the street drug market from either gateway drugs such as cannabis, i.e., marijuana, or from prescribed opioid drugs such as fentanyl, and began a very difficult road that became a hard one to exit. The feeder pathway needs to be included in community discussions. It needs a seat at the table of resolution. Part Two of this book addresses the challenges from many views and repeats important points to invigorate readers by reinforcing their internal belief that they will achieve freedom from dependency, addiction and use through personal empowerment and commitment.

Chapter One: The Scope of the Problem

The prevalence of opioids witnessed a significant shift, accounting for a mere two percent of identified addictive substances in 2014, surging to nine percent by 2018. Even after adjusting for delayed reporting, the projected number of drug overdose deaths exhibited a modest increase of 0.5% from the 12 months ending in December 2021 to the same period in December 2022, rising from 109,179 to 109,680.

Notably, the most substantial percentage surge in overdose deaths in 2022 was observed in Washington and Wyoming, where fatalities rose by 22%. In North America, fentanyl plays a dual role. It is utilized as an adulterant in various drugs such as heroin, cocaine, and methamphetamine, and it is employed in the production of counterfeit pharmaceutical opioids. Additionally, there is emerging evidence suggesting the injection of stimulants into illicit opioids. These are new influences at work, new and unknown dangers with which to cope... the balance of use to need, along with government's responsibility to address alliances and force them to curtail and end the avalanche of fentanyl and opioids' into the country has been destroyed. We are threatened by the power of the drugs, by the pharmaceutical companies and the cartels that produce and distribute them because we and our government have allowed their power to be such a threat. Our communities and citizens have lost confidence in the government.

In the past two decades, there has been a marked escalation in opioid prescriptions, leading to a surge in opioid addiction, hospitalizations, misuse, overdoses, and fatalities. This prompted me to delve into the symptoms indicative of what I may say is overuse, dependency and addiction, as well as the general hurdles and risks associated with myself and others developing opioid addiction and use disorder (OUD) among chronic pain patients undergoing chronic opioid therapy (COT).

Prescribed Addiction

One often overlooked factor driving the fentanyl and opioid epidemic was the emergence of a new market: the chronic pain pharmaceutical market. Before the epidemic, there was no dearth of opioids for acute pain. In fact, back in 1980, acute pain was so often treated with opioids that propoxyphene was the second-most dispensed prescription drug in the United States. The Carter White House declared, "Diversion, misuse, and abuse of legal drugs may be involved in as many as seven out of ten reports of drug-related injury or death".[1] But, non-cancer chronic pain was managed largely with cognitive behavioral therapy, even hypnosis. Pain advocates began to recommend opioids for chronic pain on a long term basis. Addiction was not a concern due to a pair of influential studies that found little evidence of risk.

Dependency and addiction to prescribed fentanyl and opioid pain medication nevertheless followed and grew due to the reality that individuals like you and me develop a physical and/or psychological reliance on these drugs fairly quickly. Dependency or addiction can begin within the first two weeks of use. Dependency occurs when the body adapts to the presence of the medication, leading to tolerance and withdrawal symptoms if the drug is discontinued abruptly. Addiction involves a compulsive urge to use the medication despite negative consequences, such as impaired functioning, health issues, and social problems. Both dependency and addiction can and do result from legitimate medical use of opioids, as well as from misuse or abuse of these medications. Many times the feeder process moves the prescribed patient into the use of the illicit or street drugs that have had serious consequences on our society.

Self-Cured Addict

Why did addiction take hold of me? Were there viable alternatives available? Why wasn't I adequately informed about the risks and dangers of fentanyl and other opioids and provided with options for alternative pain relief methods? These are questions you may have and that demand personal reflection and assessment. Similar to my experience, you'll likely discover that the roots of your fentanyl / opioid use, dependency, and addiction that reflect the crisis gripping our nation, are multifaceted.

According to the *New England Journal of Medicine,* the surge in prescriptions for opioid analgesics stands as a primary driver of addiction. The report highlights a staggering quadrupling of opioid prescriptions between 1999 and 2010. This surge was primarily fueled by the widespread use of opioids for pain management, coupled with a lack of recognition by prescribing physicians regarding the associated risks of opioid use. Opioid misuse is growing as a national crisis, costing an estimated $2.5 trillion between 2015 and 2018 in increased medical spending, lost productivity, lives lost due to overdoses, and more.[2]

> *"God [is] faithful, who will not suffer you to be tempted above that ye are able; but will with the temptation also make a way to escape, that ye may be able to bear [it]." Cor 10:13*

Self-Cured Addict

There can be no doubt that prescription opioids can be an important tool for managing pain; yet, improper prescribing, and the failure to properly oversee the short and long term use including excessive dosages or extended use[3] has been an important contributor to the opioid crisis, and numerous state and federal efforts have been launched to alter physician prescribing practices.[4] In my exploration of my own needs, I uncovered the significant role of prescription opioids in fueling the national crisis. Several studies underscore a compelling point: merely receiving a prescription for an opioid is correlated with heightened rates of persistent opioid use and subsequent healthcare encounters related to opioid misuse. This fact gains even more gravity when we consider the potential complications that may arise if one encounters the Coronavirus. It's a sobering reminder that when grappling with chronic pain and the consequences of opioid use, careful consideration is essential. In summary, we know very little today about the differential impact of regulations on patterns of opioid and non-opioid analgesic use for those with and without chronic pain. The responsibility simply lies within ourselves to establish a strong working relationship with our physician to monitor medication and to identify points that suggest we as patients need to address the timely and managed ending of use.

Self-Cured Addict

Before accepting your physician's recommendation, it's crucial to arm yourself with questions about treatment options, success rates, and both short-term and long-term risks, including the risk of dependency. It's also imperative to inquire about the physician's plan or timeline for discontinuing the use of these medications.

In my research, I encountered troubling reports indicating that prescription opioids often serve as a feeder process, the gateway to heroin or illicit fentanyl and opioid use. Reflecting on my own experience, I recall how I felt increasingly reliant on pain relief, leading me to hoard opioids for a rainy day. The thought of being without those pills or patches was daunting, and I can empathize with how dependency and the potential lack of prescribed drugs could drive a patient to seek alternative, often dangerous, options. This feeling led me to plan for purchasing street drugs in replacement to pending decisions by my physician to stop renewing my prescriptions.

It's true that opioid prescribing rates have declined since their peak in 2010, yet they still remain elevated compared to rates in the 1990s. Moreover, prescription opioid analgesics continue to be implicated in over a third of all fatal opioid overdoses, with the remainder attributed to heroin and illicit fentanyl. These sobering statistics underscore the urgency of addressing the opioid crisis and exploring safer non-pharmacologic patient centric alternatives for managing the immediate and defined long term use of fentanyl and other opioids in the management of chronic pain.

Under the oversight of the AMA[5], doctors are increasingly motivated to adopt a more cautious approach to prescribing opioids. Embracing a "patient-first" philosophy, physicians should prioritize ensuring that patients have a comprehensive understanding of and agreement with their prescribed treatment plan. This entails a concerted effort to reduce prescriptions for opioids or refrain from prescribing them altogether whenever feasible, while adhering to a stricter, more justified prescribing standard, particularly for high-risk patients.

For individuals coping with chronic severe pain, opioids may represent the only viable solution for achieving relief and maintaining functionality in daily life. Similarly, for patients experiencing acute severe pain, such as post-surgery or trauma, a short-term course of opioids may be instrumental in facilitating healing and recovery. In these scenarios, the potential benefits of opioid use must be carefully weighed against the associated risks. It's imperative that physicians initiate discussions about the eventual discontinuation of opioid therapy, even at the outset of treatment. Clinicians, physicians and other healthcare providers require enhanced education and training to effectively assess, treat, and monitor patients with pain, especially those who "require" and are prescribed opioid analgesics. Recognizing the limitations within the healthcare system, I assembled a small team made up of my wife, my pharmacist and physician to collaboratively manage my care. While there is a growing trend towards reducing opioid prescriptions, it's essential to strike a balance and to avoid an overly cautious approach that may inadvertently restrict access to opioids for patients in genuine need of pain management support.

"Out of 89 million opioid prescriptions issued between July 2012 and December 2017 study period, of which nearly 11 million were new prescriptions."[6]

Not all opioid prescriptions are inherently inappropriate. Assessing the appropriateness of opioid therapy hinges on accurately gauging the severity of pain, which can be challenging for prescribers without a standardized measure. Nevertheless, prescriptions carrying a high risk of misuse or inappropriate use require careful scrutiny and intervention to mitigate potential harms associated with opioid pain medications. Striking a delicate balance is essential to safeguard against misuse while ensuring access to appropriate pain relief for those who truly need it.

If you find yourself grappling with chronic pain and your primary care physician is unwilling to consider opioid therapy, even with a mutually agreed-upon treatment protocol, it may be beneficial to seek guidance from a pain specialist and secondary opioid from a different physician. Drawing from my own experience, I recommend initiating a pre-prescription appointment with your personal physician for a discussion to anticipate how the physician might approach your specific condition and treatment needs. This proactive approach can foster a more productive dialogue and potentially lead to a more tailored and effective pain management plan.

An intriguing discovery I made is that individuals hospitalized with opioid addiction or opioid use disorder (OUD) may encounter overt discrimination when they are denied access to post-acute[7] care facilities. This finding is what caused me to resolve to self-manage my way free from addiction with the oversight of my physician.

In 2018, researchers reported that out of 2,190 hospitalizations associated with addiction / OUD, 1,648 resulted in referrals to 285 facilities. Shockingly, 81.8% of these referrals were rejected. More than one-third of hospitalizations (37.4%) experienced at least one opioid-associated rejection, with 15.1% of all rejections being truly discriminatory. About three in ten facilities (29.1%) had at least one discriminatory rejection based on opioids. These statistics are not only interesting but also deeply concerning for those of us seeking to reclaim our lives and break free from addiction. This reality reinforced my resolve to self-manage my tapering process without additional medications. By taking control of your journey in a similar manner, you can avoid encountering such unacceptable treatment.

Moving forward, it's imperative for prescribers, pharmacists, and patients to collaborate closely to ensure that patients' pain management is regularly reviewed and conducted safely. Prescribers and pharmacists need to enhance their ability to identify patients who are at the highest risk and provide them with informed guidance on utilizing resources like the FenBlock and its associated process, alternative medications, addiction counseling, and other interventions aimed at facilitating tapering off medications as swiftly as possible.

There is a compelling case for future research to examine the frequency of inappropriate opioid prescribing among patients transitioning from hospitals to skilled nursing or rehabilitation facilities. Additionally, a reevaluation of prescribing practices within hospitals and their subsequent outcomes, particularly as patients transition back home from skilled nursing or rehabilitation facilities, is warranted. Such studies can offer valuable insights into optimizing pain management practices and minimizing the risks associated with opioid use and misuse.

In the 2024 PA and Yale[8] study, researchers analyzed data collected from 1,958 people who participated in a prior study by Yale and University of Pennsylvania researchers (called the Yale-Penn study) of substance use genetics.

The study's researchers examined the role of recently developed inherited risk scores for opioid use disorder and environmental and psychosocial factors such as education level, adverse childhood experiences, and related psychiatric conditions. The findings, published in *Psychological Medicine*, showed that environmental factors explained more risk for opioid dependence than did inherited risk scores. Selected environmental factors, such as annual household income and education level, explained on average three-fold greater risk than the opioid use disorder polygenic risk scores alone.

The study also found that among people with higher opioid use disorder polygenic risk scores, those with higher education level were less likely to have opioid dependence, whereas those with post-traumatic stress disorder (PTSD) were more likely to have opioid dependence than those without PTSD.

I am convinced through my own experiences that there exists an excessive reliance on opioids across various pain management approaches, undoubtedly serving as a primary catalyst for the widespread "epidemic" of prescription opioid addiction and abuse that may also feed the acquisition and use of illicit drugs throughout the United States. As a post-surgical cancer patient, the most critical personal revelation I had was that I wasn't initially accountable for my addiction. However, I've come to acknowledge that as a discharged patient, I was sitting on a ticking time bomb.

It's tempting to attribute blame to the original prescribing physician or even to the personal physician overseeing my pain management, especially if discussions regarding the need to taper off medication were lacking. The pharmacy and pharmaceutical company could also be targets for criticism, particularly if adequate guidance on tapering protocols was not provided within the drugs' FDA required instructions for use.

Research conducted by the National Institutes of Health (NIH) and the Centers for Disease Control and Prevention (CDC) underscores the concerning repercussions of prolonged prescribed opioid use. Such extended usage can according to their studies result in significant nerve damage across various muscle tissues, and vital organs like the brain, lungs, and heart. Consequently, this damage can impair the body's ability to produce natural pain-relieving endorphins, culminating in an inability to effectively regulate or alleviate pain.

National Survey on Drug Use and Health 2016, 11.5 million people misused prescribed opioids. An estimated 91.8 million adults used prescribed opioids without realizing addiction risk.[9]

Furthermore, the nerve damage inflicted on vital organs like the heart and lungs due to opioid, including fentanyl use heightens the susceptibility to severe complications from COVID-19 or possible future viruses. This increased risk is attributed to the weakened condition of these organs resulting from opioid-induced damage. Moreover, the persistent degeneration of nerve cells responsible for naturally mitigating pain can precipitate an irreversible physical dependence on opioids. Abrupt cessation of opioid use may trigger withdrawal symptoms, including sweating, insomnia, and nausea, as the body endeavors to restore balance following prolonged exposure to opiates.

No matter how good your intentions are, they amount to nothing if you fail to take the necessary steps to make them happen.

The quest to end addiction, particularly to potent drugs like hydromorphone and fentanyl, delves deep into the intricacies of the brain. Recent findings published in *Science Magazine* suggest that addiction may stem from genetic variations that influence dopamine regulation, consequently reshaping the brain's neural pathways. Understanding how addiction alters the brain's dynamics prompted me to confront the challenge of overcoming addiction while managing underlying pain.

One hallmark of opioid addiction lies in the euphoric and dissociative experiences induced by dopamine release upon drug consumption. Left unchecked, this sensation can foster further addiction, leading to recreational or illicit drug use and heightened dependence. Reflecting on this phenomenon brought back memories of my college biology classes, where I learned about epigenetics—a process whereby inherited traits are influenced by external factors, distinct from alterations in DNA sequencing. This complex interplay of brain activity underscores the long-term ramifications of addiction, not only for myself but also for others grappling with addiction. Relating to my initial use of morphine and the years of opioid and fentanyl for pain management, I cannot recall any euphoric feelings.

Serotonin and dopamine, prominent neurotransmitters, play pivotal roles in psychological disorders like depression, anxiety, and addiction, further highlighting the intricate workings of the brain and the imperative of finding safe methods to break free from opioid addiction and related medications.

"I was shocked by the dramatic genetic altering risk addiction presents, but to act on it, I first had to decide to end my growing dependency before it was too late."

Recognizing opioid dependency hinges on identifying the telltale signs of withdrawal, a hallmark of opiate detoxification. Personally, and perhaps resonating with others, I began to experience these symptoms consistently, surfacing mere hours after each dose. This relentless pattern signaled my body's increasing demand for medication, a stark indicator of addiction that I could no longer ignore.

In hindsight, these early warning signs of dependency or addiction often go unnoticed or brushed aside as expected. Yet, they serve as crucial signals, urging individuals to embark on a journey toward tapering off opioids rather than succumbing to escalating dosages or frequency of use. It's a pivotal moment to engage in dialogue with your healthcare provider, charting a course toward liberation from addiction.

The majority of addictive substances, including opioids, trigger a surge in dopamine levels, fostering a chemically induced sense of reward that fuels intensified drug cravings. This altered reward circuitry may contribute to the profound stages of depression I endured, shedding light on why individuals grappling with depression often resort to self-medication through increased opioid dosages or why they seek out illicit substances in a bid to elevate dopamine levels.[10] Addiction, in its complexity, reflects a transformative landscape in our comprehension of the mechanisms underlying the effects of these pain management medications.

There is heightened concern and long-term risk specifically tied to women who maintain their use of opioids for pain management during pregnancy, including medications prescribed for addressing opioid use disorder. It is imperative that pregnant women reliant on prescribed opioid pain management medication engage in discussions with their healthcare provider. They should contemplate, and their doctors should encourage, tapering their dosage and with close monitoring by their obstetrician, family physician, or midwife at the initial prenatal consultation. At the very least, integrating this information into the prenatal record can mitigate risks associated with unforeseen delivery complications, including preterm birth. *Women's Health*[11] magazine provides new insight into how pregnancy and parenting can make getting medications for opioid disorders particularly difficult. According to a new study led by Penn State researchers, they may face unique challenges accessing treatment.

The researchers found that among pregnant women, common barriers to receiving medication treatment included doctors' hesitancy to prescribe these medications to pregnant patients; limited access to resources in rural areas; and difficulty navigating complex, decentralized health systems.

For women who already have children, the researchers found that a lack of childcare during appointments and meetings, fear of losing custody of or access to their children, and prioritizing their children's needs above their own were common obstacles to accessing medication.

Kristina Brant, assistant professor of rural sociology in the College of Agricultural Sciences and co-author of the study, said the findings underline the complex challenges facing these women and their children—including how the fear of losing custody of their children can prevent mothers from seeking treatment, which ultimately can be harmful for children over time. Recent studies published by the Mayo Clinic report studies performed to date have not demonstrated pediatric-specific problems that would limit the usefulness of the Duragesic® patch and Fentanyl extended-release patch in children two years of age and older. However, pediatric patients must be opioid-tolerant before using a fentanyl patch. Safety and efficacy practices however have not been established in children younger than 2 years of age. The point of the report in my view is always address your concerns through your pediatrician and validate answers as necessary. A patient is opioid-tolerant if oral or injected opioids have already been used for severe pain or if an injectable opioid has been used for sedation or anesthesia.

"It's important to design systems that prioritize families' needs and allow mothers to seek help while not fearing that it will cause a severing of their relationships with their children," Brant said.

Ultimately, this will also ensure that children get the services they may need as well." Medications used to treat opioid use disorder (MOUD)—such as methadone and buprenorphine —have been shown to be effective at reducing overdose deaths and improving quality of life generally, the researchers said, and are considered safe to take during pregnancy.

But the researchers added that in 2021, only 22.1% of people with opioid-use disorder across the country received these medications, suggesting there are barriers in place preventing both men and women from receiving care.

Abenaa Jones, Ann Atherton Hertzler Early Career Professor in Health and Human Development and principal investigator on the paper, said that while obstacles exist for people of all genders, women may experience unique difficulties.

"Previous research has illustrated that women who use drugs have different needs than men who use drugs—often centered around gendered responsibilities such as child-rearing, parenting and childcare," Jones said. "We wanted to examine this among women who use drugs and have a history of criminal legal involvement, as well as professionals who work with affected women, to develop multifaceted solutions to engage women in substance-use treatment."

For the study, the researchers interviewed twenty women who have lived with an opioid-use disorder, ten criminal justice professionals who have worked with women with opioid-use disorder and twelve substance-use disorder treatment professionals who have worked with women who have received MOUD. I noted throughout the report that having treatment facilities and programs geared towards women with children, supporting the expansion of programs geared towards mothers and their kids could help increase pathways to care. So as we move forward together we must insist that a broader approach to care is provided to protect women and children. This includes removing the stigma and challenges that women face being unable to bring a young child to an inpatient facility that today presents a huge deterrent for a mother who is contemplating seeking treatment.

I agree with the findings that punitive barriers to treatment must be removed to alleviate mothers' fear of losing custody of their children. This change would not only reduce instances of child maltreatment but also make it easier for women to seek help without facing judgment.

Parallel to the general challenges of women that I report here are the challenges facing women in criminal justice system pretty much guaranteeing them being less likely to receive treatment for opioid use. Thus the challenges for women are wide and need to be addressed.

In a January 10, 2024 news release, the NIH-supported findings suggest the need to expand definitions of addiction treatment success beyond abstinence. The report also noted that reducing stimulant use was associated with significant improvement in measures of health and recovery among people with stimulant use disorder, even if they did not achieve total abstinence. I believe this finding strongly supports my conviction that by gradually and carefully reducing the dosages of opioids through the structured approach of FenBlock, I achieved the same results that the study has now validated many years later. Historically, total abstinence has been the standard goal of treatment for substance use disorders. However, these findings support the growing recognition that a more nuanced perspective on measuring treatment success may be beneficial.[12]

Self-Cured Addict

"The only person you are destined to become is the person you decide to be."
—Ralph Waldo Emerson

NIDA Director Nora Volkow, M.D. said in the study: "Embracing measures of success in addiction treatment beyond abstinence supports more individualized approaches to recovery, and may lead to the approval of a wider range of medications that can improve the lives of people with substance use disorders." This is a supportive statement to the process of graduated tapering that is the basic technique employed with the help of FenBlock.

Further according to the study; "With addiction, the field has historically acknowledged only the benefits of abstinence, missing opportunities to celebrate and measure the positive impacts of reduced substance use," said Mehdi Farokhina, M.D., M.P.H., a staff scientist in the NIDA Intramural Research Program, and author on the study. "This study provides evidence that reducing the overall use of drugs is important and clinically meaningful. This shift may open opportunities for medication development that can help individuals achieve these improved outcomes, even if complete abstinence is not immediately achievable or wanted."[13]

My goal is to help you along with all patients and doctors, understand the risks associated with current abstinence-based opioid treatments compared to a more logical and graduated approach like FenBlock. It's crucial to have a thorough understanding of these risks so that patients and supporting physicians can make informed decisions that minimize the likelihood of relapse.

There is special concern and long term risk specifically associated with women who continue their use of opioids for pain management while in pregnancy. This includes medications prescribed for addressing opioid use disorder. All pregnant women reliant on prescribed opioid pain management medication need to discuss their situation with their physician. Once FenBlock has been approved by the FDA, they should consider reducing their opioid pain medication through the device's graduated barrier approach and request that they be closely monitored by their obstetrician, family physician, or midwife at the first prenatal consultation.[14] At a minimum, having this data as part of the prenatal record will reduce risk associated with unexpected challenges in delivery including preterm birth. Symptoms of opioid withdrawal can be unpleasant, but they are generally not life-threatening. However, when symptoms include vomiting and diarrhea, they may lead to severe complications such as dehydration due to fluid loss and reduced sodium levels in the blood. Opioid withdrawal can also trigger suicidal thoughts and ideation, which can potentially result in death. Undergoing recovery from opioid addiction under medical supervision at a treatment center or through self-empowered tapering with medical oversight significantly reduces these risks. Establishing and adjusting your own timeline as needed, and adhering to your tapering process, will also minimize risks while empowering you to achieve success.

> *"The most common way people give up their power is by thinking they don't have any."*
> —Alice Walker

As you progress through your tapering process and begin to decrease your dosages, you may encounter some of the following common withdrawal symptoms:

- Mental reminders or cravings to return to previous dosages or restart opioid use altogether

- Decreased feelings of nausea as withdrawal progresses
- Elevated blood pressure
- Stomach cramping
- Sweating
- Chills or goosebumps
- Diarrhea
- Irritability or agitation
- Anxiety
- Muscle aches
- Shakes or trembling
- Insomnia
- Dilated pupils
- Spending less time with friends and family
- Prioritizing opioid use above hobbies, interests, and responsibilities
- Quick, lightning-type striking pain

Prescription opioid addiction can affect anyone. It's crucial for you and your physician to closely monitor your medication and recognize signs of dependence on opioids and to recognize the point where tapering off your drugs is necessary. Additionally, monitoring your emotional state and identifying any compulsive urge to continue using or increase dosage is essential and for the same purpose. Despite attempts to quit and awareness of the negative consequences of opioid use, you may still feel the need to use them. Collaborating with your physician or medical team ensures that all risks are addressed and mitigated effectively. We have underused treatments that could help many people. We must meet patients where they are to prevent overdoses, reduce harm, and connect people to inviting means of solution treatments like FenBlock to reduce and end drug use while mitigating their risk of withdrawal.

> *"It is the strong in body who are both the strong and free in mind."*
> —Peter Jefferson, the father of Thomas Jefferson

Globally, approximately 35.6 million individuals grapple with opioid and drug use disorders. Although opioid usage is more prevalent in developed nations than in developing ones, the affluent segments of society exhibit a higher prevalence of opioid use. However, individuals who are socially and economically disadvantaged are more susceptible to developing opioid use disorders.

Unfortunately, only one out of eight individuals in need of opioid-related treatment actually receives it. Despite the fact that one out of three opioid users is female, only one out of five individuals in treatment is a woman. Moreover, individuals in prison settings, minorities, immigrants, and

Self-Cured Addict

displaced persons encounter obstacles to treatment due to discrimination and stigma. These barriers exacerbate the challenges in accessing essential care and support for those struggling with opioid use disorders.[15] Simply increasing access to clean needles, fentanyl test strips and Naloxone, a drug used to rapidly reverse opioid overdoses is not the total answer. The feeding pattern of drug abuse needs serious examination, discussion and corrective attention.

An analysis of statistics from the US Centers for Disease Control and Prevention, used to declare that prescription opioid abuse had reached epidemic levels, reveals that addiction, abuse, and deaths are increasing outside the hospital setting, implicating the outpatient use of opioids to treat chronic pain, as in my case. It is evident that addiction, abuse, and related deaths occur among chronic pain patients. Using data from the 2013–2017 Medicare Part D database, I found: The average number of opioid prescriptions per beneficiary (OPBs) decreased from 1.08 in 2013 to 0.87 in 2017. There were several factors associated with a higher OPB, including a younger population, higher education levels, and higher health care costs. Counties across the country with fewer mental health providers and higher uninsured rates also saw higher OPBs. "In my study, we were surprised by the variance of opioid prescription rates across different states." These facts can be important to remember and, where appropriate, to point out during conversations with your physician. An informed patient or patient's advocate is incredibly helpful when it comes to managing your use away from addiction to its end and regaining your freedom.

As soon as FenBlock is approved by the FDA and is available, individuals like you and me will be in position to make the decision, with your physician's oversight and coaching, to break free from opioid dependency and use. It will be possible for you, as in my case, to become rehabilitated, freed from addiction and drug use, whereas the evils of fentanyl, opioids, and other narcotics have no chance for rehabilitation. People using drugs are not the evil component. In instances where addressing pain is imperative, it becomes crucial as you focus on ending your use and dependency on addictive medication to explore managed tapering using non-opioid and non-medicated solutions as viable substitutes. Addicted or dependent individuals fall into two categories, lost and unchangeable apathetic, or passionate and seeking life's goods. Depriving the power of drugs [evil] in our body with their self centered instincts and idolatry that replaces our devotion to God will bring true freedom from addiction and return the glory to God. I prefer to focus on passionate acceptance and love in order to encourage those lost to join us anytime.

Opioids, including fentanyl, stand as effective medications integral to well-rounded multimodal pain management strategies for acute pain in postoperative patients. However, the equitable distribution of pain relief medicines remains a global challenge. In 2018, over ninety percent of all pharmaceutical opioids designated for medical use were concentrated in high-income countries. North America accounted for fifty percent, Europe forty percent, and Oceania an additional two percent—despite these regions representing only about twelve percent of the world's population.

Thus there is a stark imbalance to the urgent need for concerted efforts to ensure equitable access to effectively managed pain relief medications worldwide. As access is expanded, it is imperative to establish standards requiring appropriate prescription and physician oversight and management, ensuring responsible patient usage and tapering where necessary.

Barriers to accessing pharmaceutical or prescribed opioids are influenced by various factors, encompassing federal and state legislation, prevailing cultural norms, the structure of our health systems, and adherence to professional prescribing "best practices."

As you reflect on my narrative of opioid addiction and my empowerment to self-managed care, should any immediate questions arise, I encourage you to engage with your physician or personal healthcare provider promptly for directive coaching. Seek their guidance or reach out to the U.S. Substance Abuse and Mental Health Services Administration (SAMHSA) National Helpline at 1-800-662-HELP. Take the precautionary step of entering this information into your phone for quick access. Your proactive approach to seeking assistance when needed is vital.

My story, much like yours, is authentic and profoundly personal. Yet, akin to allegories, it possesses the potential, and I fervently hope, the capacity to enact transformative change. Such metamorphosis can be sourced from a myriad of inspirations, including some of the most foundational inquiries in philosophy.

Consider Plato's allegory of the cave, Montaigne's musings on the nature of existence through the lens of a cat, Kierkegaard's daring leap of faith, and Nietzsche's profound myth of eternal recurrence. These intellectual companions stand poised to accompany us in our quest to unravel the intricacies of addiction, relapse, and recovery.

In weaving together our personal narratives with these profound philosophical insights, we embark on a journey of exploration and understanding, seeking not only to comprehend but also to transcend the complexities that tether us to the struggles of addiction and the promise of freedom from our use of drugs.

Find Your Courage Through Faith

My surgery and later addiction captured my resolve to face my state of cancer and future use through my faith in God's words. The Bible emphasizes the importance of self-control and sober-mindedness (1 Peter 5:8, Galatians 5:22-23). I knew my substance abuse impaired my judgment and self-control, which could lead to harmful behaviors. I knew the Bible encourages believers to find comfort and strength in God during times of difficulty rather than to seek escape through substances (Philippians 4:6-7). My knowledge that Christians are encouraged to take care of their bodies (1 Corinthians 6:19-20) and avoid anything that would harm them gave me the strength and hope that I would achieve my return to good health and freedom from my use of drugs.

And let us not grow weary of doing good, for in due season we will reap if we do not give up.
—*Galatians 6:9*

Individuals such as you and me struggling with addiction to substances like fentanyl or other drugs can find guidance and support in these biblical teachings on sobriety, self-control, and seek help and redemption through faith and community. The study of Simon, also known simply as Peter, played a role in my decision to end my use. Peter was one of the twelve apostles chosen by Jesus Christ to be his closest follower and disciple. Peter is often depicted as a prominent figure among the disciples, known for his passionate devotion to Jesus, his leadership within the early Christian community, and his role as a key witness to Jesus' ministry, death, and resurrection. Simon Peter exhibited human weaknesses and struggles as well, such as his denial of Jesus before his crucifixion. Peter's story can serve as a testament to the transformative power of faith, forgiveness, and redemption, illustrating how even those who falter, such as you and me, can be used by God to accomplish great things.

It's important to note that I understand the Bible does not explicitly mention addiction in Peter's life. Nevertheless, his experiences offered by biblical historians put forward valuable insights and lessons for me and indeed for everyone grappling with the challenge of addiction. Through Peter's example, individuals like you and me can find encouragement to seek appropriate treatment and healing (James 5:14-15) by relying on faith, and striving for personal growth and transformation.

Self-Cured Addict

Peter was a prosperous merchant known for his wealth and influence in the community. His story indicates he harbored a secret struggle—one that threatened to consume him entirely. Peter had fallen victim to the allure of opium, a potent substance much like fentanyl and opioids today that promised fleeting relief from the burdens of life. What had begun as a means of escape from the stresses of his daily endeavors had spiraled into a crippling addiction, clouding his judgment and enslaving his soul.

> *1 Peter 5:8, "Be alert and of sober mind. Your enemy the devil prowls around like a roaring lion looking for someone to devour."*

As Peter's addiction deepened, so too did its impact on the community, and it became reflective of today's epidemic. Families were torn apart, livelihoods were lost, and the fabric of society began to unravel under the weight of addiction's grip. Despite the growing devastation wrought by opium, many turned a blind eye, choosing to ignore the plight of their fellow brethren rather than confront the harsh reality of addiction. Within this story I found myself many times returning to prayer for strength and commitment to end my addiction and regain freedom from drugs.

But amidst the darkness, a voice emerged to Peter—a prophet named Elijah who spoke with unwavering conviction and compassion. Elijah bore witness to the suffering inflicted by addiction and called upon the people to heed the cries of the afflicted. He implored them to cast aside their indifference and extend a hand of empathy and support to those ensnared in the throes of addiction.

Inspired by Elijah's message of hope and redemption, I too was inspired by God's words. Simon's community, like my community of family and friends, rallied together, united in their resolve to confront the scourge of my addiction head-on. Through education and outreach efforts, Simon sought to raise awareness about the dangers of addiction and break the cycle of silence and stigma that shrouded the issue.

Over time, Simon found the courage to confront his addiction and to seek help in order to regain his life. With the unwavering support and the guidance of compassionate mentors, he like me embarked on a journey of healing and transformation. Through faith and perseverance, Simon emerged from the depths of addiction, renewed in spirit and purpose.

As the sun set on the land of my home in Forest, Virginia, a new dawn of hope arose—a testament to the power of faith, compassion, and solidarity in overcoming addiction's grip. The story of Simon served as a poignant path for me and a reminder of society's collective responsibility to address addiction with empathy, understanding, and unwavering resolve—together, and bound by faith, love, and compassion, we can overcome even the greatest of challenges. Facing the challenges brought on by addiction, we all need to refer to stories of redemption, forgiveness, and spiritual transformation, from which you as I did will find hope and strength in your journey toward recovery and healing. While the Bible may not directly address our modern drug challenges, its teachings emphasize the importance of caring for our bodies, exercising self-control, to help us find strength and solace through God, rather than turning to substances for comfort or escape.

It is my prayer that my story will strengthen your commitment to safely ending your use, dependency and addiction. I welcome you sharing your path with me as I will retain you in my prayers. Joy is a choice to trust His faithfulness, even when the path ahead is unclear.

Chapter Two: Reflections

In Part One of this book I explained how I was able to free myself from addiction to fentanyl. Once FenBlock is approved and you embark on this path, I suggest you maintain a detailed log of your reductions and document your physical and emotional states on a daily basis. Throughout the initial month, the second month, and beyond, you'll be able to compare your progress and recall your observations at each interval. Feel empowered to make additional notes to affirm your ongoing progress or signal the need to adjust your pace. Remember, the decision lies entirely with you. Should you encounter obstacles or bottlenecks, don't be deterred. Instead, pause to assess the situation, restructure your plan, realign your priorities if necessary, and reset your target dates to resume your journey towards freedom from addiction.

The satisfaction derived from this process is truly profound, so embrace it wholeheartedly. You can achieve this, and if you require assistance along the way, don't hesitate to reach out. I am committed to providing whatever support you need. As a fair-minded individual, my goal is to help safeguard your life and enhance the lives of those around you. Freedom, my friend, is a shared priority for both of us and for everyone on your support team.

Self-Cured Addict

When I freed myself from hydromorphone, for example, I meticulously documented each step of the pill shaving and chipping process, retaining the fragments as evidence until only a sliver remained, signaling the end of my medication intake. The success of my journey can be attributed to the gradual and manageable tapering process, coupled with the absence of significant adverse reactions. While I did experience minor headaches, occasional vomiting, and periods of depression, I deemed these to be minor compared to my previous experiences before tapering. Remarkably, as I tapered off the powerful opioid, these symptoms lessened. Despite the underreporting of suicides in opioid-related poisoning deaths, I never entertained thoughts of self-harm or suicide. However, I advise against immediately subjecting yourself to such risks. Should you find yourself grappling with such thoughts, reach out without delay to your practitioner and trusted family, friends, and faith leaders, your moral shareholders. A deeper understanding and improved assessments of emotional well-being, particularly concerning suicide risk in patients with pain and those taking opioids, are imperative.

Having successfully tapered off hydromorphone, my next challenge was discontinuing fentanyl, a significantly more potent and addictive opioid. Tackling this task presented daunting hurdles. Initially, I grappled with devising a strategy for tapering off the fentanyl patch, a unique challenge given its design. Unlike pills, the patch couldn't simply be cut or folded to adjust dosages.

Recognizing the necessity for patients to gradually reduce fentanyl intake from the patch, I sought an impermeable barrier of suitable size, adjustable to accommodate the desired percentage of reduction. This level of control and adaptability formed the foundation of what evolved into the FenBlock.

Fentanyl is a synthetic opioid agonist that interacts primarily with your mu-opioid receptor. The low molecular weight, high potency and lipid solubility of fentanyl make it suitable for delivery by the prescribed transdermal therapeutic system. These patches are designed to deliver fentanyl at a constant rate (25, 50, 75 and 100 mcg/h), and require replacement every three days. Transdermal fentanyl is effective in the treatment of chronic cancer pain. No obvious differences in health-related quality of life were found in patients with chronic cancer pain when comparing transdermal fentanyl with sustained-release oral morphine. Because of the formation of a fentanyl depot in the skin tissue, serum fentanyl concentrations increase gradually following initial application, generally leveling off between 12 and 24 hours. Thereafter, they remain relatively constant, with some fluctuation, for the remainder of the 72-hour application period. Once achieved, steady-state plasma fentanyl concentrations can be maintained for as long as the patches are renewed. Fentanyl taken orally must pass through the lining of the digestive tract presenting risks of serious digestive tract pain and disruptions through its direct impact or interference with other oral medications. Based on my experience and given the drug's absorbability in my digestive track, I experienced severe abdominal pain, and I was switched to the fentanyl patch transdermal delivery process.

Understanding the associated risks should be a collaborative decision-making process between patient and physician or healthcare provider long before the patient needs to choose the most suitable treatment for chronic pain. Opioids serve as reliable medications that alleviate pain, enabling individuals to find relief before and after surgeries and other medical conditions that induce varying levels of pain over various periods. However, alongside providing pain relief, opioids can also induce sensations of feeling good, even euphoria, which contribute to the development and perpetuation of addiction.

Self-Cured Addict

"Opioid addiction is very much still an empirically driven discipline and the FenBlock is setting out to change that - and formalize the individual's role."

Opioids pose a significant risk of addiction due to their ability to bind to receptors in the brain, triggering sensations of reward and euphoria. Misuse of opioids, especially in high amounts, can lead to fatal overdoses. On a daily basis, the opioid epidemic claims the lives of over one hundred fifteen individuals in America due to drug overdoses. This statistic encompasses both street opioids like heroin, as well as prescription opioids administered by healthcare providers. Over the past decade, opioid overdose deaths in the United States have surged, now standing at five times higher than they were just a decade ago. The misuse of opioids not only imposes substantial healthcare costs on the nation but also results in significant lost productivity for businesses and profound disruptions to countless families across the country.

"Together you the reader and I are on a quest to uncover a more natural, objective way to cure addiction, self-determination."

Now that the medical community is encouraging physicians to cut back on prescription narcotics, the addicted patients in concern for their physician's ending prescription renewals are turning more to readily available alternatives such as street heroin and fentanyl as I was preparing to do. The fear of withdrawal symptoms and craving for the drugs were so intense that they kept me on a continuous search for more opioids.

Progress is evident in the fight against the opioid use, misuse, addiction crisis. For instance, there was a notable thirteen and a half percent decrease in prescription opioid-involved overdose death rates from 2017 to 2018. Moreover, encouraging trends in addiction and opioid abuse rates have been observed across various demographics, as reported by the HHS and CDC:

- Across the age group of fifteen to sixty-four years
- Among non-Hispanic Caucasians, Hispanics, and non-Hispanic Native American Indian/Alaskan populations
- Across all levels of urbanization
- In seventeen states, there has been a decline in prescription opioid-involved overdose death rates
- While stable in the Northeast, rates have decreased in the Midwest, South, and West regions

The National Institutes of Health notes that prescription

opioids were once considered non-addictive as long as they were used to manage pain, leading to an increase in prescriptions and subsequent dependence, illicit opioid use, and fatal overdoses. Recognizing the severity of the crisis, the federal government has declared the opioid epidemic a national public health emergency, prompting a comprehensive and collaborative effort to address the issue.

> *"The [opioid] crisis is a formidable challenge that's rapidly evolving, so our research response has to match both in magnitude and in urgency," said HEAL Initiative director Dr. Rebecca Baker*

Individuals who use prescribed opioids for genuine medical reasons may inadvertently develop a physical dependence on these medications. Shockingly, over forty percent of overdose deaths in 2016 were attributed to prescription opioids[16]. This statistic underscores concerns about the United States' prescribing practices, considering that while it comprises only five percent of the global population, it consumes a staggering seventy-five percent of all prescription drugs manufactured worldwide.

Initially, when my physician discussed the post hospital treatment plan for my chronic pain condition, I felt well informed and believed he had my best interests at heart.

However, with the increasing attention on prescribed opioid addiction and misuse, and its feeder patterns that can result in transitioning to street drugs, I have gained a deeper understanding of the risks involved. Armed with this knowledge, I made an informed decision to confront and overcome my addiction before I would obtain street fentanyl and opioids to fill what I feared to be on the horizon, my physician's refusal to refill my prescription. The fear of not having the drugs was at times overbearing and placed my mind in a very dangerous place. It was only through prayer that I maintained a sense of responsibility to not further endanger myself.

An educational strategy targeting providers, patients and payers, is needed to connect and to create better pain care and timelines to end unnecessary addiction before it starts.

Addiction to prescribed opioids, as highlighted in a 2019 issue of the *New England Journal of Medicine,* can develop alarmingly quickly, sometimes within just two weeks of the patient's initial use for severe or chronic pain treatment. This startling revelation underscores the origins of the addiction crisis, which partly stemmed from physicians being misled in the early 2000s about the low risk of addiction associated with prescribing opioids for chronic pain. Moreover, an earlier study published in June 2017 by the in the prescribing of potent opioids like oxycodone, hydromorphone, and fentanyl over the past two decades. The NEJM also reported a staggering toll of deaths attributed to prescription opioids in the United States alone, with millions more Americans falling into addiction through the prescription process. Lost within the prescribed world of addiction became a daily theme, which is reflected in the following narrative:

Opioid Use Disorder care is delivered in silos, rarely coordinated or comprehensive, focusing on treatment not cure.

In the serene hush of a morning much like today, I confronted the pressing urge to extend beyond my prescribed doses of fentanyl and opioids. Just as today, the community's struggle with prescribed fentanyl / opioid users slipping into street drugs lingered beneath the surface, camouflaged amidst the daily reports of illicit fentanyl-related fatalities linked to cartel-produced substances amid the broader epidemic of addiction. Yet, I found myself ensnared in the street addiction labyrinth due to a flawed prescription oversight and control system. As the roots of my addiction evolved into street supply considerations, that insatiable appetite for more began to assume more personal control. Seeking refuge in my supply, I scoured the streets and witnessed the effortless accessibility of fentanyl, morphing it into a conduit leading to street fentanyl,

Self-Cured Addict

cocaine, or heroin. I stood on the brink of becoming another statistic, had it not been for my turning to God.

> *"I am the vine; you are the branches. If you remain in me and I in you, you will bear much fruit; apart from me you can do nothing."*
> *John 15:5*

Reflecting on God's poignant words in John 15:5, likening Him to the vine and us to the branches, I am reminded of the profound significance of my connection to Him for my very existence. Today, as a recovered fentanyl addict, I have embraced this truth and forged a path towards a richer, more fulfilling life. This verse beckons us to scrutinize our relationship with Christ. Are we drawing our strength and sustenance from Him? In moments of despair, when the weight of addiction and the clamor of need seem insurmountable, it is within this divine union that we discover the capacity to flourish and bear fruit that mirrors His love and character. Through Him, like me, you can break free from the grip of addiction with the support of others. You are not alone. By remaining rooted in Jesus, grounded in His teachings and love, we not only survive but thrive, producing fruit that enriches the lives of others and glorifies God. What steps can you take today to deepen your connection with Jesus? Draw strength and guidance from Him. Seek counsel from family, friends, as well as our dedicated police and medical professionals. God is ever-present, ready to embrace us all.

In addition to the need to advocate for more prudent opioid prescribing practices and reducing prescriptions where feasible, there's a glaring lack of momentum toward finding a cure. While opioids offer essential relief for some patients suffering from chronic severe pain, such as in my case, the destructive impact they can and have had often goes undetected. Over the seven years of my prescribed hydromorphone, hydrocodone, and fentanyl regimen, I remained oblivious to their potential harm, a sentiment no doubt shared by many readers.

Despite the vital role opioids play in managing acute pain, particularly post-major surgeries or trauma, there remains a concerning absence of guidance on mitigating addiction risks and implementing effective tapering strategies to empower and invite users to turn to ending their use. While my doctors were forthright about the benefits of opioids during periods of acute pain, they never broached the topic of tapering, ending my use, nor did they provide comprehensive information on the associated risks that I retained by continuing my use. This simply needs to change through a better dialogue between patient and physician that sets a meaningful objective to address pain and monitor the person's performance to acknowledge a time when ending their use is identified.

It's crucial for practitioners to receive enhanced and continual education on assessing, treating, and monitoring patients with pain, especially those prescribed opioid analgesics. This needs to be patient-centric and responsive to their concerns over the stigma associated with addiction and the potential for success in their freedom from addiction and overall use. Primary care providers often lack sufficient training in these areas, leading to these gaps in patient care. Many states have acknowledged this deficiency and mandated additional training as part of licensing requirements.

Furthermore, the Food and Drug Administration (FDA) has recognized the imperative for prescriber education and, since 2012, has mandated that opioid analgesic manufacturers offer unrestricted grants for continuing education providers to develop training aligned with the FDA's Opioid Analgesic REMS Education Blueprint for Health Care Providers Involved in Pain Treatment and Monitoring.

Self-Cured Addict

True treatment efficacy hinges on patient centric, user self-empowerment and ownership of one's addiction journey. Without embracing our capacity to end addiction through coaching focusing on self-empowerment self worth, the risk of relapse or tapering failure looms large. The path to curing opioid use disorder (OUD) begins with acknowledging our addiction, accepting our agency in ending it, and recognizing that each step in our individual process contributes to a successful self-managed cure.

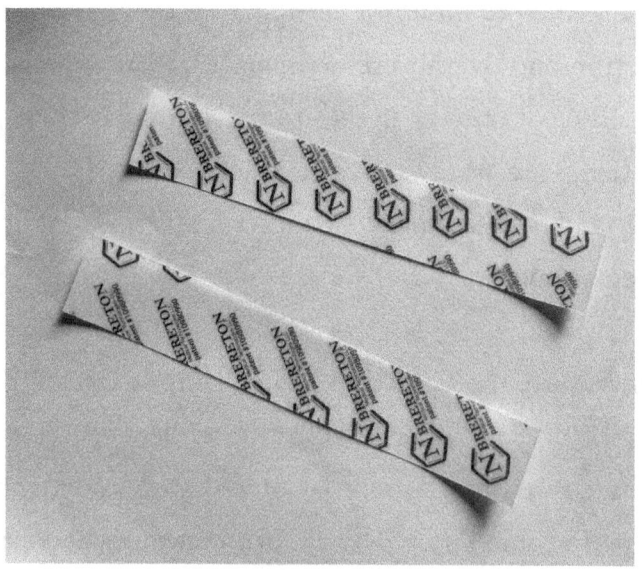

FenBlock™

Patent No. – US 10,661,065-B1; US 10,842,980-B1; US 10,980,990-B1

Chapter Three: Pain & Addiction

How many of us have peered into the mind of an addict? How many of us actually conceive their situations, understand their weakness in motivations and address how they and their method of use can be solved? I will attempt to reveal the answers and present sound arguments for the reader to make the decision for themselves, or for others they love to regain their health and hope for life. My true story is non judgmental in scope and firmly grounded in the fundamental principle that embracing a life with Christ can be a beacon to guide you and to empower you to effectively conquer addiction. As the Lord said, we shall be called to a greater work, he also asks, "Have you done what you could? Not for yourself, but for others?" I believe the focus on ending drug addiction should not be through speech, it ought to be through action, new techniques, and new options, and new products such as FenBlock.

Pain was the last thing I wanted from the surgery, and it was the first item to be addressed by the hospital via a morphine drip immediately after surgery. My journey with pain, and possibly yours as well, began being treated immediately with opioids.

Self-Cured Addict

Dr. Hornicek expressed astonishment that a sixty-one-year-old could endure such an extensive operation aimed at removing an eight-and-a-half-pound tumor in one piece. Upon my discharge in August 2012, I was prescribed nine-hundred milligrams of Gabapentin to be taken four times daily, alongside thirty-two milligrams of hydromorphone administered at 8:00 am, 4:00 pm, and 10:00 pm plus. However, the heavy dosage of hydromorphone soon led to erratic swings in comfort, accompanied by spikes in intestinal pain, headaches, and severe nausea.

Soon after release, and in response to these problems, my physician made adjustments to my pain management regimen in mid-2013, introducing a transdermal patch of one-hundred microgram (mcg) of fentanyl through the transdermal patch to be replaced every seventy-two hours. While initially successful in masking the pain, my brain presented escalating demands for greater relief, which became apparent by mid-2014, causing significant distress. After careful consideration, my physician opted to increase the frequency of the one-hundred mcg fentanyl patch application from every seventy-two hours to every forty-eight hours.

Given the unprecedented complexity of my surgery and subsequent pain management, both my physician and I navigated uncharted territory, learning from each other's experiences. Despite my routine consultations with the prescribing physician at MGH, discussions rarely broached the topic of asking about my [growing] opioid dependency, now recognized as prescribed opioid addiction. Instead, the consensus reaffirmed my status as a lifelong chronic pain patient, with minimal alterations recommended to my treatment plan.

As the torchbearer of future prescribing decisions shifted to my personal physician from MGH, I grappled with the realities of managing chronic pain and the associated risks of opioid misuse, abuse and dependency.

"If conscience errs resulting in steps back not forward, shake off ignorance, with grace regain dignity before blinded by habit."

As I'm sure you realize, amidst the journey, I've gleaned invaluable insights that I'm eager to share, particularly regarding my strides toward reclaiming independence and freedom from addiction. Research from the Oregon State University College of Pharmacy underscores a concerning trend akin to my own experience. It revealed that hospital patients discharged to skilled nursing and rehabilitation facilities, as I was when I was moved to their Spaulding Rehab Center, often carry high-dose painkiller prescriptions with them. While my transition to MGH's long-term rehabilitation center was seamless, it sheds light on the need for heightened patient-centric attention to opioid safety and encouraging subsequent tapering upon transfer and discharge.

This pattern mirrors the challenges faced by low-income Native American populations, who endure higher rates of pain and comorbidities with limited access to pain management resources, including non-pharmacological treatments. The disparity underscores the urgency for a more comprehensive approach to opioid and fentanyl safety and management, particularly in vulnerable populations and transitional care settings.

It is in witness to and appreciation to the God who has given rebirth to my life, and now awaits you, that I want to encourage you to do what you can to end your use of these drugs and to recapture and strengthen your love for God, life, health, hope, and freedom from addiction. When you begin with gateway drugs or opioid pain medications, transitioning to illicit drugs can be compared to exchanging a handgun for a machine gun. Through the lens of a patient-driven, non-pharmacological approach, it highlights the pivotal role spirituality can play in addressing and ending opioid addiction without any gun to your head.

Observe, Understand, Accept, Act

I want to confront the fact that Narcan is the new device to carry for saving the lives of a user's error or an addict's misuse or overdose. It encapsulates a pivotal chapter in my life, akin to a curtain call—an encore after the performance of overcoming severe addiction that spanned seven challenging years. Much like a performer yearning for the continuation of their act, it was through my expertise in the taking of drugs that afforded me tremendous insight and credibility from which I was awakened and sought an extension of my life. I asked questions about the options society has, including government-provided, that I could use to play a significant part in controlling my destiny. Sure I was an addict. I had ceded control to drugs in exchange for perceived comfort. I witnessed the congruence of government policy [politics] and healthcare were off target for what I saw as needed. The options were limited to alternative drugs or rehabilitative services or the use of brain modulation, both of which would leave me without any control—a state I'd lived in for years, and control was something I wanted desperately to recapture. From the pantheon of government experts, scientists and private practice physicians and psychiatrists, the limited "solutions" were void of the patient's or user's experiences and needs, and hidden from them were the risks.

I did not desire to contradict my God-given will to live by not acting. I knew deep inside I could end my use, but the avenue to do so had to provide me time, flexibility and empowerment if I was to succeed. Throughout this journey of discovery, my wife Darlene, our children, Neil Jr. [Brett], Devon and Laura, as well as friends served as my unwavering and encouraging audience. It is my hope that through my experiences previously described in Part One that you too will find the strength and decide to taper off your use, eventually to achieve full recovery and happiness.

I recognize the fentanyl crisis is a tremendously complex public health issue and have deep sympathy for everyone affected, which is why I am working to expand new innovative technologies to help those in need solve their addiction.

In Luke 16:8 Jesus reminded me that "the children of darkness [me the addict] are wiser than the children of light."
This gave me strength.

Self-Cured Addict

Looking back, my nightstand was covered with bottles of prescription drugs. Reported daily in the news were the growing problems of opioid addiction, overdoses and fentanyl deaths. Our governor and his attorney general crisscrossed the state expounding on the evils of street drugs and cartels in our towns and cities while the government legalized marijuana sales and use without speaking honestly of the reality that it can be a gateway drug that leads to illicit street drugs. My cause was real. My brain, my body signaled my craving for comfort and protection from pain. My brain swung widely from engagement to doubt, to fear, to depression, to nausea, to anger without hesitation and sometimes it came close to the thought of suicide. I was living a life long sentence of dependency in the "management of pain."

Being in the situation I was in, you see huge mountains looming, and you start wondering how you are going to scale those heights, end your dependency, your addiction and your drug use. Because you are not looking where you are going, you stumble on the easy path where I am leading you now. As I help you get back on your feet, you remember how worried you are about the cliff up ahead. Will freedom from addiction be on the other side? God and you alone know that it will. In you with Him exists the power to hope and achieve freedom from addiction. Remove yourself from the stigma of use. You have God. Perseverance is His charge to you. He has equipped you with the tools for your climb, your ascendence to freedom.

As you now know, my story of triumph began with my battle against severe addiction, triggered by the aftermath of cancer surgery. It commenced innocently enough with a morphine drip, evolving into the administration of oral opioids, and eventually culminating in the heavy prescription of various opioid medications, including the potent fentanyl patch, all aimed at masking the chronic post-surgical pain.

This narrative unfolded beyond the confines of the hospital, extending unchecked through my release and the subsequent seven years of difficult physical healing and recovery. From the pronouncement that I will be a chronic pain patient for life, thereby justifying my use of narcotics I asked myself, had I been deceived? And if so, by whom, my physicians, the hospital, and my pharmacist? Have I been ignorant and unwilling to seek help? The answer to all is no. The crux of my journey and possibly yours with all its threats and uncertainties led me to a profound realization. Faced with the choice of perpetuating a life tethered to dangerous medications, marked by experiences of near death depression, nausea, and migraine headaches, or summoning His strength within me and the encouragement of my family and friends to embark on a path to freedom, I reached a critical juncture.

Assuming Fenblock is approved, it will be important for you to consult your physician or a healthcare professional about any concerns on FenBlock graduated tapering plan options, dosing, or any other questions relating to FenBlock and other N Brereton Medical Technologies products.

In a landscape where discussions often center around prevention, treatment options, and support, it is high time to shift our focus towards effective cures and innovation in solutions. We need action. This narrative unfolds as a testament to human resilience and underscores the significance of patient preference, innovation, and desire.

My personal journey compelled me to embrace patience, innovation, invention, fortitude, and self-empowerment in my quest to conquer opioid addiction and reclaim freedom. The chosen path paved the way for a restorative blueprint—a cure that will extend its potential to millions grappling with a variety of opioid addictions. While my emphasis lies in the realm of prescribed opioids, the core principle of self-empowerment, deeply ingrained in the fabric of America's culture, and the invention of a graduating barrier tapering technology holds promise for addressing a spectrum of drug addictions for others.

As my personal journey attests to the effectiveness of this process and invention of the FenBlock barrier technology and device in facilitating my recovery, I am unwavering in my conviction that my story and resolute focus on self value represent a secure and winning solution for others. This approach not only provides a practical avenue for addressing prescribed opioid and fentanyl addiction but also offers a viable strategy for combating societal stigma, and pressure to seek treatment or change behavior before reaching legal or life threatening consequences.

According to the Centers for Disease Control (CDC,) anyone who takes prescription opioids can become addicted to them within two weeks. In fact, as many as one-in-four patients receiving long-term opioid therapy in a primary care setting struggles with opioid addiction. In December of 2018, when the CDC declared fentanyl the deadliest drug in America, I was already six years deep into what I call overuse and a severe addiction involving the highest prescribed dosage of fentanyl and other opioids. The pivotal role of pre- and post-surgical prescribed opioids in shaping my personal crisis and contributing to the broader national epidemic became evident, placing patients at an elevated risk of persistent [after prescriptions expire] opioid use without an anticipated timeline for use or physician followup. As an addict of prescribed opioids, the intrinsic threat of misuse or denial for drugs never deflated. As mentioned, I anticipated my physician's refusal to renew my prescription and began hoarding pills and patches for a "rainy day" while being fed to and looking for street alternatives. I'm no different than anyone in the same situation, one you may be in as well. I hope through my story the light of hope comes on and you too choose the path to your successful end of dependency and use, your return of freedom and health.

It took more than seven years before I challenged my fentanyl and opioid medication dosages. Had I heard earlier from my physician, or a friend or family member who was concerned that I was addicted and wanted to help, I may have taken action before and saved years of suffering from the impact of the drugs. If you know or think someone is struggling with addiction, I suggest that you ask them if you can help. Your concern might be what is needed to start their tapering and recovery journey. Your support could make all the difference in their success.

My profound realization stemmed from the recognition that prescription opioids had unwittingly paved the way for potential progression towards illicit fentanyl and other potent narcotics such as heroin and cocaine. It was much too late into my struggles when I grasped the harsh reality that there was a void in my discussion with my doctors and pharmacists about prescribed opioids as gateway drugs to more dangerous substances. Thus, what began as a simple press of the morphine button for pain relief gradually spiraled into a relentless demand for drugs, not for euphoric purposes but simple internal demand evolving into a full-blown addiction. The signs of addiction were unmistakable: escalating doses, stockpiling for future use, and frequent refill requests. Despite those glaring red flags, I remained unchallenged, and my drug consumption continued unchecked.

Have you ever pondered the decision to change course, wondering what your experience may be, or if your experience may mirror mine? Have you felt concerned about the drugs and the doses you've been taking or using? Have you explored the idea of altering your path and putting an

Self-Cured Addict

end to your usage? Are you worried about the lingering pain, discomfort, depression, or withdrawal symptoms? These were all considerations that crossed my mind, and I'm confident they cross your mind, too. However, without a clear reason or incentive to end my seven-year dependency, I found myself stuck in acceptance of my situation. Neither my physician nor my family and friends had offered any persuasion for me to consider a different approach. To be honest, I never reached out because I felt my use was just fine. The turning point in my journey to overcome addiction arrived shortly after the President of the United States announced the formation of the Commission On Combating Drug Addiction and The Opioid Crisis in 2017, casting a spotlight on the severe opioid epidemic afflicting the people of our nation. This announcement sparked a series of personal reflections and inquiries. I found myself questioning why I remained reliant on these drugs despite several years passing without follow-up from my initial prescribing doctors regarding tapering off. I delved into understanding the factors that led to my addiction and pondered how I would feel once I discontinued fentanyl and other opioids. Concerns about potential health consequences and injuries to my major organs, including my brain, loomed large and prompted me to expand my investigation efforts. Moreover, I wondered why alternative non-opioid pain relief or pain management options weren't presented before my release from the hospital. The President's announcement addressed the pressing need to address the opioid crisis in the United States, and it challenged the nation to provide novel ways to combat drug addiction and the opioid epidemic, including strategies for prevention, treatment, and recovery. Its aim to encourage development of solutions and recommendations to help tackle the growing problem of drug addiction and overdose deaths across the nation motivated me to seek answers to these initial concerns, although I grappled with worries about the timeline and the process. I also fretted over how my physician would react to my desire to end my usage, fearing that he might find reason to not renew the prescriptions without providing a transitory process. Despite the negative thoughts swirling in my mind about ending drug use, my determination to break free had been awakened.

The literature I encountered, which remains the same today, failed to illuminate the long-term risks and intricacies of quitting, leaving my journey, much like many others, devoid of insights into the subtle signs of addiction and methods to break the brain's demand for these drugs. The demand was simple to understand. My brain told me I needed more—an incredible but true statement. After the initial morphine button, there were no euphoric feelings. I only felt secure if I had enough to keep me going. I worried about not being able to fill a prescription when I was out of town. As you know, prescriptions for controlled substances are not easy to transfer from one pharmacy to another. So, I hoarded pills and patches. I began to get prescriptions filled early. Over years I hoarded hundreds of hydromorphone and gabapentin pills and over seventy fentanyl patches. I had found a method of increasing my use without asking my physician for more. I realized at the end of my tapering process that the process was enabled by the fact there was no follow-up, no advice by a physician concerning the option of tapering off. Like many, I placed trust in the physician's guidance. Now, with hindsight, I trust in tact in direct relationships and communications between physician and patient.

Embarking on a reflective journey of my experiences, I am happy to have shared the empowering story of how I navigated a mission that could potentially ignite the courage needed to reassess reliance on prescribed or illicit opioid pain medication. Coming from a situation that may be just like yours, I hope my narrative has and will serve as a compelling beacon for individuals grappling with opioid addiction, offering them the resilience to confront and triumph over their challenges. The road ahead may appear daunting, dotted with obstacles. Yet, I can affirm that maintaining a positive and self-empowering attitude, bolstered by the support of faith, family, and friends, will fortify your resolve every step of the way.

> *And let us not grow weary of doing good, for in due season we will reap. if we do not give up.*
> *—Galatians 6:9*

Drawing from my path, my aim is and has been to transmit and instill the resilience required to retrospectively evaluate my recovery from surgery to unequivocally decide that "enough is enough." Despite exhibiting no overt signs of opioid use, earning compliments from doctors for enduring substantial opioid volumes—a lingering sense of vulnerability persisted.

The President's Commission's report prompted a transformative shift in perspective on that pivotal day. As previously mentioned, I found myself engrossed in C-SPAN as the Attorney General and President addressed the nation's opioid epidemic. It was a moment akin to gazing into a mirror; a profound realization struck me—I knew by the grace of God they were speaking directly to me. This seemingly inconspicuous yet potent juncture marked an irreversible turning point in my life. Having not only endured but triumphed over the formidable challenge posed by the intense opioid dosages I had consumed, I now perceive it as my duty to share my story and to underscore the methods through which I conquered addiction.

The crux of future solutions in pain management, as you will come to appreciate, lies in the advocacy for and enforcement of judicious opioid prescribing with strict practices for physician follow-up and improved controls over dispensing prescription refills aligned with insurance payment practices. The imperative is clear: to actively identify, promote, and implement measures that curtail unnecessary opioid prescriptions and renewals wherever feasible.

Recognizing the imperative need for positive changes in prescription policies amid the U.S. opioid epidemic, it becomes crucial to augment patient data to guide doctors in identifying moments when patients should gradually reduce and ultimately discontinue reliance on and use of opioid medications. Currently, the absence of an accurate method for measuring pain compels patients, including myself, to often declare the highest levels to secure maximum medication. Adding that to the absence of a sound system of controls over the insurance payer system, we have enabled corruption by the patient through misuse of a weak system.

It is essential for both the FDA and all healthcare providers to reevaluate protocols concerning an accurate assessment and measurement of pain, and to establish clear standards to ensure accurate long-term evaluations. This step is essential in fostering awareness and promoting responsible management of fentanyl and opioid prescriptions after hospital discharge. Its absence reflected a major failure in my case.

Once approved, a method such as the utilization of Fen-Block and its processes will offer to those addicted or dependent a viable option to safely taper off their usage and regain their health. Although the journey may be with imperfections, it holds the potential to be transformative, enabling informed decision-making and the establishment of personalized timelines on the path to freedom. The Fen-Block barrier technology will provide individuals with the flexibility to articulate their goals, set timelines, and make necessary adjustments with their physician's oversight, all with a focused commitment to the long-term elimination of use.

Self-Cured Addict

I trust you find it enlightening and empowering.

"I will give you a new heart and put a new spirit within you and I will remove the heart of stone from your flesh and give you a heart of flesh. And I will put My Spirit within you and bring it about that you walk in My statutes, and are careful and follow My ordinances."

—*Ezekiel 36:26-27*

Chapter Four: Face the Facts

Throughout my journey I told myself to trust in God and His forces that are so much greater than mine, forces wise and good that shape each day. I am not one who reflects on a lot of things. But what I went through was a lesson in reality few have ever experienced. What did I learn? There is always right and wrong. Simplified things are not simple. The research I did to learn about myself and fentanyl and other opioid drugs that were prescribed, was to help me determine the best and safest method of getting off those drugs. I read, prayed, and thought about things.

What brought me to the point of knowing that I must persist and find a cure? Looking back at my life's journey, who had the greatest influence? No doubt it was my mother, Marjorie E. Jackson, a care giving nurse who in my youth as I had dealt with multiple surgeries had always been my light of hope. She knew and reminded my brother and me every day why God created us—to know, love, and serve him. She was a Red Cross Volunteer nurse, always there when trouble impacted others. She was our mom when trouble impacted us. How then did I end up with a prognosis of chronic pain and lifetime assignment to powerful life threatening, life changing opioids? What had I learned through my mom in those earlier times that I

Self-Cured Addict

could use? I needed to learn even more and to understand. Opioids were new to me, and I knew I needed to learn their potential for good and bad. Would every day with chronic pain and its relief through opioids be the same or would the days be different?

I learned in school a very important rule that I used in the hospital: never skip over a word that you read or heard that you do not know. My research showed that the history of fentanyl began in 1960 with a Belgian chemist, Paul Janssen, who pioneered the synthesis of the opioid fentanyl[17], a morphine-like substance. Historical accounts highlight its revolutionary impact on surgical anesthesia and postoperative pain medication. Fentanyl, boasting a potency 150 times greater than morphine, marked the inception of a new opioid family for human use, and I would experience its good and its bad. Like all narcotics, fentanyl, a great pain reliever, carries with it significant risks. Administration in sufficient quantities can lead quickly to addiction, respiratory and mental depression, hypoxia, a reduced heart rate, and, in extreme cases, death. I would learn to take longer views, to prepare for the rainy days, to prepare for the unexpected future, to think ahead and not to expect gratification. Maybe not knowing is actually an advantage because throughout my journey I saw life in a totally different way. It was not rosy. Pain and its relief from drugs had started something I did not and could not control. How would I control the consequences? I would soon learn. Should I tell people to leave me alone, that I prefer to make my own decisions, or do I reach out to those I love for help, to my faith for strength? Did they see what I would become?

The National Institutes of Health reports that over eleven percent of adults in the United States grapple with chronic pain. In the pursuit of enhanced pain management, there was a notable four-fold surge in opioid prescribing, culminating in the onset of an opioid epidemic. In 2015 alone, in the middle of my misuse and addiction, a staggering 12.5 million individuals misused prescription opioids, resulting in over 33,000 deaths from opioid / fentanyl overdoses[18].

> *A record number of Americans died from drug overdoses in 2021 as the powerful opioid fentanyl continues to fuel a national drug crisis. Overdose deaths involving opioids such as illicit fentanyl and heroin jumped from an estimated 70,029 in 2020 to 80,816 in 2021.*[19]

Opioid addiction presented heightened concerns, especially as the nation continued to grapple with the Wuhan COVID-19 epidemic, and at the time of this writing, it prepared for the "next pandemic." If you find yourself addicted to fentanyl or other opioids, whether for pain relief or other reasons, your vulnerability increases in the event of contracting COVID-19 and possibly other viruses yet to be faced. COVID-19 slows your heart and breathing rate and when combined with the use of opioids which act in the same manner, your risk of serious consequences, including death, would likely be proportionately higher. These circumstances underscore the urgency for you to make the decision to timely taper off fentanyl and all opioids, not only to overcome addiction but also to enhance your overall survivability, particularly in the face of the COVID-19 or a similar virus threat. What I saw by examining the nation's addiction challenge was a nation driven by "effort justification." Take for example our current state, as I write this, of open borders and its impact on addiction and death of Americans while the government remains a promoter of their efforts to end addiction's scourge against America and the destruction of the American family.

In my quest to end addiction, I encountered a significant gap—a lack of publicly available methods or devices that offered a definitive path of low risk to a potential cure for my placement drugs, brain / sound modulation systems, but no comprehensive risk measured cure. I found no solution that encouraged me to try something I could measure and manage and partner with my physician in order to totally end my use.

The FenBlock barrier technology and supporting process stands apart by not relying on addiction rehabilitative treatment, substitute medication, risky brain modulation or recent invasive probes into the brain to correct receptors and end the feeling of addiction. Understanding that a component of opioid and fentanyl addiction begins with prescribed medications, there needs to be a realization that prevention of illicit drug addiction needs to include the application of FenBlock barrier technology to help prescribed users end their use before they enter the illicit street market. FenBlock doesn't necessitate admission to rehabilitation. Rather, its focus is on enabling those who wish to take steps to cure themselves to do so, albeit with the oversight and coaching of a physician. The objective is to harness inner strengths, leading to the elimination of prescribed or illicit opioid medications, as well as to the improvement and reclamation of damaged relationships, all with the ultimate goal of recovering and enhancing an individual's happiness.

Self-Cured Addict

"Be watchful, stand firm on the faith, act like men, be strong."
—*1 Corinthians 16:13*

"I can do all things through Him who strengthens me"
—*Philippians 4:13*

In moments of uncertainty regarding your addiction, embrace the truth about yourself without fear. Seek external perspectives from your faith, loved ones, friends, your medical practitioner and care team.

"Be courteous to all, but intimate with few, and let those few be well tried before you give them your confidence."
—General George Washington

Whether you are using prescribed or illicit drugs, the same necessities can apply to you. Through this exploration, which occurs with self-awareness, you'll realize that awareness of your support to help end your addiction and use extends beyond yourself. Embrace your inherent fearlessness to fortify your resolve. Take this book and apply its practices to reassess your perception of addiction, and your inner strength for securing your path to freedom from its grasp.

Self-Cured Addict

OPIOID related inpatient hospital stays INCREASED 117% nationally from 2005 to 2016.[20]

Navigating life with opioid addiction often leads us into the realm of self-denial. I, too, resisted acknowledging my addiction, merely continuing with the "pain" medication. Addiction, however, is indiscriminate, affecting people across all backgrounds—regardless of emotions, achievements, financial status, or poverty. Succumbing to self-denial won't liberate you from addiction or restore your freedom. It's merely another detrimental choice.

Breaking free from addiction will serve as a testament to your inner character's resilience and empowerment, propelling you towards victory. My story recounted in Part One encapsulates my journey of self-empowerment and faith in God triumphing over prescribed opioid addiction. Thankfully, it occurred before I would inevitably have entered the street illicit market to feed my growing demands. I am confident it can become your story of triumph as well. I pray that it will.

Commencing with the origins of my addiction, its gradual evolution over seven years, and culminating in my triumphant conquest by drawing upon the pillars of faith, family, and my moral compass, while steadfastly upholding my need for wisdom, integrity, truth, and character as my ultimate rewards of reclaiming freedom. Personal autonomy is integral to my comfort, as I am not inclined to relinquish control over my decisions, health, or daily activities to others. I believe these feelings and deep beliefs are within us all. Determined to find the most effective method under my sole control, I embarked on a quest for options and a "best-of-breed" approach to safely, without residual pains or withdrawal, and no recidivism, to terminate my seven-plus year addiction to potent opioids—hydromorphone and fentanyl.

Thoroughly researching my complicated addiction opioids, while anticipating potential challenges in the cessation process, I was totally disappointed that there was no acceptable option. I meticulously devised a twelve-month tapering plan. I believed setting the timeline initially at twelve months was reasonable. I knew that as a self managed process, along with my physician, I could change the timeline as needed, by shortening or lengthening it based on the results I recorded during the tapering process. This plan, designed with minimal risk (non intrusive, non-pharmacologic and without rehabilitative services), and with my physician's participation, served as my guide from the initial day of tapering until the pivotal moment of "kicking my addiction" on the last day. The key reason to avoid rehabilitative services was my reluctance to "surrender personal control" to practitioners who know nothing about me including my personality. Plus rehab is expensive and the warranty on its success is less than desirable. I had previously given up the self control points during the eleven months at Massachusetts General Hospital.

> *Self-love requires that you never permit any*
> *abuse upon yourself or others.*
> *There is no virtue in allowing abuse.*

However, the unknown variable was how to implement the tapering process, involving opioids [34 mg of hydromorphone pills, 24mg of gabapentin, and a one-hundred mcg[21] fentanyl patch], and then determining how it would impact the recurrence of chronic pain or result in any form of withdrawal. The uncertainty of whether pain would manifest immediately, over time, or not at all compelled me along with my concern of withdrawal challenges to embark on a unique, graduated tapering plan, fully aware of the potential mental, physical (pain), and emotional reactions that might unfold. I say unique because I was unable to find any similar "safety net" type of approach. I decided at the same time to create and maintain a diary of sorts to log the daily activities of the tapering timeline.

Self-Cured Addict

My medication regimen, consisting of two distinct delivery methods—pills and patches—necessitated tailored steps and different tapering devices for each. Taking charge of my tapering mission, I recognized the importance of formulating reasonable processes that were achievable. While acknowledging the potential need for adjustments based on personal feelings, locations, and unpredictable [previous] results, I valued the flexibility provided by having control over FenBlock's graduated tapering barrier amounts and procedures. Would I increase or decrease the barrier size? I knew I needed the ability to do both. This autonomy allowed me to promptly respond to the emergence of pain or other withdrawal symptoms, which I never experienced (and to which I give praise to FenBlock) without seeking agreement with or permission from others for temporary dosage increases. From the onset and throughout the tapering process I kept my physician informed and we routinely met for discussions on status and any adjustments as needed. I urge you to set up the same framework. Once approved, doctors will be provided with information about Fenblock as well as recommended coaching and oversight steps.

Initiating the tapering process, I began by consulting with my family physician to discuss my plans for ending the addiction, expressing my concerns, outlining the proposed reached an agreement that I would keep him informed of my steps and progress. Establishing a written log for each step as I noted earlier, and documenting any reactions, we decided that I would promptly notify him of any challenges or withdrawal effects that occurred. This collaborative approach transformed our physician-patient relationship into a partnership. My physician became my coach. Recognizing the evolving nature of this partnership, I believed that having greater self control over the pace of reduction provided me the freedom to modify my timeline based on the reactions to tapering off the drugs. Again, this was done with the physician's total awareness.

Embarking on my mission, I extensively searched the Internet for successful articles, delved into medical journals, and explored addiction research reports and stories centered on tapering practices and results. Despite my efforts, I encountered surprise and disappointment as I failed to find any accounts or methods detailing a successful and low-risk process for gradually tapering off opioids in a safe, and managed way. What was I going to do?

My primary goal was to liberate myself from addiction without experiencing adverse effects such as withdrawal symptoms or heightened pain. Given the dual nature of the

Self-Cured Addict

opioids I was taking, I recognized the need for two distinct tapering processes. Opting for simplicity and safety, I decided to initiate the tapering process with the pills[22].

As you read in Part One of this book, for hydromorphone, also known as Dilaudid, with was prescribed in non-extended release pill form, I devised a method involving a pill slicer to chip away very small pieces. This gave me the ability to test the reactions of my body and brain. Initially, I took a minimal chip off one pill on the first day. Over the course of a few days, I gradually increased the size of the chipped portion from one pill. Throughout this process, I meticulously maintained my written log, recording the approximate amount chipped off, and stored the pieces in a plastic sandwich bag for verification. This tapering process spanned nearly seven months. As I approached the end of the timeline, the remaining chip from the last pill was so small that I decided to conclude my dosage by pill. By the conclusion of the hydromorphone pill tapering, the sandwich bag was half full. The process at the beginning was "trial-by-error" and by the second month it was a formula that built up my resolve that I had made the right decision and was proud of each day's accomplishments.

Self-Cured Addict

Throughout the chipping process and the documentation of daily, weekly, and monthly logs, I observed the continual lessening and disappearance of severe nausea, headaches, suicide level depression, and spikes of pain that had been prevalent before commencing the tapering. My friends had noticed my skin color was better. The whites of my eyes were turning to white from a yellow tint. Are these scientific findings? Not at all. They are real experiences that build resolve empowering me to continue, and that I hope and pray work for you. I regularly shared summaries of the log entries with my physician through email, webinar, or meetings in his office, receiving feedback and addressing any concerns or comments he raised.

Remarkably, I did not notice any problematic withdrawal symptoms during the tapering, and the process did not feel endless. Adhering to a bi-weekly reduction in dosages became a routine[23] that progressed swiftly. Consistent communication with my physician and pharmacist also proved beneficial, as they cautioned that despite the absence of withdrawal symptoms, opioids might have stored medication in cells throughout my system. The pharmacist suggested that it could take about three months for these stored medications to dissipate, potentially leading to the onset of withdrawal symptoms during that period. As those few months passed I did not experience withdrawal.

I did know that my drugs were "missing." But that feeling may have been a result of my own subconscious feeling. Regardless I was not uncomfortable mentally or physically at any point. Overall, I was excited and proud. My physician was in disbelief, having never seen a patient do this.

Having successfully concluded the tapering process with hydromorphone pills, I now turned my attention to the fentanyl patch—a distinct form of opioid delivery that required a unique approach. Fentanyl patches contain fentanyl in two layers, an upper reservoir layer (containing 6% fentanyl) and a lower donor layer in contact with the skin (containing 4% fentanyl). The "liquid" within the permeable patch demanded careful research to develop a reasonable and effective tapering strategy while minimizing risks.

Unfortunately, no documented studies or clinical research provided guidance on tapering off the fentanyl patch, necessitating the creation of something entirely new.
Challenges arose due to the patch's design, which prevented folding or cutting without rendering it useless or risking excessive leakage onto the skin, potentially leading to a risk of overdose. Friends had suggested cutting the patch and resealing it with tape. My concern focused on the risk of unnecessary contact with fentanyl. Faced with these risks and constraints, I embarked on designing a so-

testing with various "non-transdermal" materials to determine its efficacy in safely tapering off fentanyl.

As you recall reading in Part One, the unique attributes and tapering challenges of the fentanyl patch compelled me to innovate and invent the FenBlock graduated barrier device, which could adjust in a graduated and managed control of the fentanyl substrate's absorption into the skin. Through an iterative testing process on myself, I identified a material that successfully halted the flow and thereby the absorption of the fentanyl substrate. After thorough personal validation and additional enhancements to the prototype barrier design, FenBlock emerged as a practical solution for me to use.

At the culmination of my extensive research, design, fabrication, testing, and validation, I achieved my goal of creating a safe, simple and scalable barrier device that is flexible to contour, adheres to the skin, and maintains the patch's integrity that can be used on any patch. Importantly, FenBlock eliminated the need to substitute tapering medications, and the need to revert to the oral fentanyl [pill], which would have presented the risk of irritating my digestive system, which had been the reason my doctor and pharmacist had switched me from fentanyl pills to the

Self-Cured Addict

transdermal fentanyl patch. FenBlock also allowed me to avoid the risk of introducing additional addictive substances or resorting to costly rehabilitation measures including device maintenance (chip, batteries, parts), invasive and high risk brain modulation devices, probes, and so forth.

Throughout my research and the progression of my timeline to overcome addiction, the inadequacy of opioid addiction solution and use disorder services in the United States remained a significant issue. It was disconcerting to discover that less than half of addicted adults were receiving tapering treatment, let alone achieving a solution, a use-ending cure. A critical observation emerged from the Substance Abuse and Mental Health Services Administration's 2018 National Survey on Drug Use and Health, involving over 65,000 respondents. The findings were troubling, indicating that only one in five individuals with an opioid/fentanyl use disorder sought any form of treatment. Maybe one reason for such an absence of support for tapering can be traced to the fentanyl patch manufacturer's instructions for use packaged with every box of patches. The instructions are extensive on placement, use, disposal, etc. while only two sentences discuss tapering off.

Self-Cured Addict

On January 10, 2024, the National Institute on Drug Abuse published "Reduced drug use is a meaningful treatment outcome for people with stimulant use disorders."[24] The study found that more participants reduced the frequency of primary drug use (18%) than achieved abstinence (14%). While abstinence was associated with the greatest clinical improvement, reduced use was significantly associated with multiple measures of improvements in psychosocial functioning at the end of the trials, such as a 60% decrease in craving for the primary drug, 41% decrease in drug-seeking behaviors, and a 40% decrease in depression severity, compared to the beginning of the trial. "This study provides evidence that reducing the overall use of drugs is important and clinically meaningful. This shift may open opportunities for medication development that can help individuals achieve these improved outcomes, even if complete abstinence is not immediately achievable or wanted." The authors highlighted that the findings of this study should encourage researchers to reevaluate treatment outcome measures in their studies and consider non-abstinence treatment outcomes in the development of new medications for the treatment of stimulant use disorders. The authors also wrote that these new findings need to be replicated in other contexts with additional substance use disorders such as opioid use disorder.

Self-Cured Addict

"And let us run with perseverance the race marked out for us."
—Hebrews 12:1

Respecting the current definition of needs by NIDA, as I viewed the need for improved capabilities, my disappointment extended beyond the limited scope of the article, which focused on addiction prevention and treatment without addressing the crucial aspects of when to address the need to graduate the tapering and ending the patch use and curing the patient's addiction.

Furthermore, the article failed to provide data on access to or an invitation for innovators to encourage emerging research and development of devices and methods for safely solving addiction. There was simply an absence of resources guiding individuals on how to find a remedy, connect with providers, foster needed inner strength, empower themselves, end any focus on stigma, and independently manage the course to taper off fentanyl and opioids. This void compelled me to "take these matters into my own hands."

The foundations of these findings and the absence of any emphasis on ending my use and achieving a solution / cure, whether medical or non-medical, are intricate. Firstly, opioid addiction or use disorder remains highly stigmatized across our nation. Many patients, myself included, face limited access to care due to:

- Cost barriers
- Uncertain limitations to insurance coverage
- Uneven geographic distribution of clinical resources
- Overall scarcity of knowledgeable trained general practitioners, and clinicians treating patients effectively with opioid use disorders
- Indigenous Nations and Tribes around the world are underserved by limited and unacceptable treatments

The restrictive nature of insurance arrangements, which I personally experienced, and the inclination of practitioners treating opioid use disorders to operate independently and inconsistently, reflected the absence of measurable standards of practice. This contributes significantly to discouraging practitioners from joining insurance networks and treating opioid / fentanyl use or addiction. This web of factors hinders the pursuit of effective, affordable, and accessible treatment for individuals grappling with opioid addiction. As a result I went to work to create and develop a simple yet powerful scalable barrier technology and a process of gradually reducing the absorption of fentanyl in order to taper off the dose of fentanyl from patches over time.

Self-Cured Addict

Overcoming the challenge of accessing available and inviting new treatments or a cure for opioid addiction or "use disorder" (OUD) faces the hurdle of denial for service by many Out-of-Network insurance care providers. This denial results in discouragement due to high out-of-pocket costs and additional barriers to treatment, which often lack the focus on a cure as the primary objective. Like many, I didn't seek mere treatment; I sought a cure.

Barriers of cost are real, and I kept this in mind as I went about the design of an affordable barrier technology. As a result, low cost became an integral requirement in FenBlock. My research uncovered no real insights into safe, graduated tapering, a process apparently not done before, and so I took it upon myself to develop one with the understanding that I would discover as I employed it myself how much tapering and at what pace I could comfortably endure. A key goal was to take responsibility for curing my addiction without relying on replacement drugs.

By taking personal responsibility I knew I needed to consult with my physician and maybe others and together to manage the process while at the same time retaining my ability to decide on options as they might occur. I sought a process surrounding FenBlock that instilled confidence and empowered me to break free permanently from the

Self-Cured Addict

Until you and I decide to reject the ideology of addictive drugs and start to live again by traditional values and faith we can never know our true value.

My afford88ability goal was achieved. FenBlock does not require entry into an expensive and control-centered treatment center. It addresses these challenges with a simple device and process that encourages self-empowerment and confidence, eliminates the need for alternative medication, eliminates unnecessary costs, and keeps an individual in the driver's seat of his or her recovery journey.

I believe it makes sense for individuals addicted to fentanyl patches and opioid pain medications to take charge of their tapering goals and timeline. In my book, it needs to be a personal choice. When considering my options, I rejected the idea of substitute drugs or third-party rehabilitation. The essential components are the patient's character, empowerment, commitment to winning, and the availability of coaching from their physician or other medical practitioners. With these qualities and access to the necessary resources, individuals can reclaim their pre-opioid life and break free from addiction.

Self-Cured Addict

In 2017, more than 11 million persons reported misusing prescription opioid analgesics during the past year, more than 2 million reported opioid use disorder, and there were, on average, 130 overdose deaths involving an opioid every day.[25]

So how do we find our national epidemic today? The American College of Surgeons reported in 2024: "It is likely that in counties with restricted health care access, due to higher health care costs, lack of insurance coverage, and decreased availability of mental health providers, patients may receive more postoperative opioids as they might not be able to easily obtain additional opioid pills should they need to, or, more likely, that the higher opioid prescribing is masking an unaddressed overall health and mental health burden in this patient population."[26] My hope is that awareness of this, if it impacts you, that you can take steps to contact your local, state and federal (www.billblaster.com) representatives to generate support for your needs. In their absence you are welcome to contact me, via the information at the back of the book.

While there are numerous self-help books, my research revealed a gap in literature focusing on opioid addiction from an independent control perspective. Surprisingly, addiction treatment-focused books do not delve into the realm of do-it-yourself (DIY) solutions. Consider this book your gateway to convincing yourself that through self-empowerment, you will be in position to overcome your opioid addiction at your own pace and under your control. Once FenBlock is approved by the FDA, FenBlock will no longer be a Do-It-Yourself process. Ending your addiction may take longer than it took to lose your freedom, but armed with the knowledge of achieving your goals through self-empowerment, freedom from addiction can become your enduring reward. The simple reasoning behind this is your will to win, your faith, and the support from your family and friends, which are significant resources to keep you on target.

The problem with prescribed opioids is that they are addictive and they kill pain – and people.

Drawing upon extensive research and personal experience, it is crucial to reemphasize that while packaged drugs contain comprehensive instructions, complete with drawings and pictures explaining how to use prescribed opioids and the associated risks to consider, there is a notable absence of similar instructions for their timely and safe discontinuance. This oversight is correctable. Also noted are the totally absurd disposal instructions. Manufacturers instruct patients to dispose of used patches by "folding the patch and flushing down the toilet." With millions of used fentanyl patches certainly with residual content of fentanyl being flushed into our drinking waters, we must demand new processes. FenBlock's disposal process includes a pre-addressed non-transdermal sealable envelope that is returned to an FDA approved medical waste company for proper incineration. I sincerely hope these practices are adopted universally.

> *"The majority of current heroin users began with prescription opioids."*[27]

During my search for alternative solutions I noted that access to residential addiction treatment centers caring for U.S. adolescents under 18 years old in the United States is limited and costly, according to a new study supported by the National Institutes of Health[28]. Researchers found currently that only about half (54%) of the residential addiction treatment facilities that they contacted had a bed immediately available, and for those with a waitlist, the average estimated time before a bed opened was 28 days. In addition, the average daily cost per day of treatment was $878, with close to half (48%) of the facilities that provided information requiring partial or full payment upfront. On average, the quoted cost of a month's stay at a residential addiction treatment facility was over $26,000. The comparative and affordable cost of FenBlock is projected to be $900 per month until an individual is free from use. When your child is in a crisis and needs treatment, it can be terrifying to know where to turn. Many parents or family members who look for residential care find the experience profoundly disheartening.

As previously stated, at the time of this writing, FenBlock was with the FDA awaiting approval. But systems-level changes that ensure effective, affordable treatment options for everyone can play a decisive role in conquering the opioid pandemic. Hopefully, this is an incentive that will result in speedy approval of the FenBlock device. You may wish to check with your physician or contact me through the FenBlock website to learn where the approval process now stands. Once FenBlock is available, a prescription by your physician is all that will be required to start you or a loved one on the pathway to freedom.

As I look at my drugs I can't explain what I'm willing to do for drugs. What woke me up is what I was not willing to become.

Chapter Five: How C-SPAN Helped

As recounted in Part One, the declaration of the 'President's Commission On Combating Drug Addiction and The Opioid Crisis[29]' served as the catalyst for me to scrutinize my reliance on pain medications. As the President of the United States and Chris Christie reported on the commission's findings, I was informed of the destruction Fentanyl and opioids were imposing on my health, and I recognized the imperative need to discontinue my use of them. During their presentation on the report and the government's renewed commitment to curbing the escalating opioid addiction and misuse epidemic across the nation, the President and Christie shed unprecedented light on the issue. Never before had such focused attention been given to the widespread use of both prescribed and illicit opioid drugs in our country. The government's strategy emphasized addressing the dual sources of addiction and misuse: the illicit trafficking of opioids, particularly fentanyl and its precursors, from Mexico, Central and South America, and China, and the prevalent prescribing of opioid pain medication in recent years.

Self-Cured Addict

"Self-pity is our worst enemy and if we yield to it, we can never do anything wise in this world."
—Helen Keller

From the stark revelations articulated that day, my resolve to break free from addiction led me on a journey to confront the unvarnished truths about the deleterious impact of opioids, systematically wreaking havoc on my health. As I absorbed their remarks, I sensed an overarching feeling that their words were directed specifically at me. At the same time, I heard a heart whisper from God that my mission was to defeat my addiction and to develop a means for others to do so as well. Their compelling presentation served as a catalyst for me to take decisive actions toward reclaiming a normal life, unshackled from the grip of addictive medications, regardless of the personal costs involved. While some may perceive this as an act of courage, I saw the alignment of choosing to watch C-SPAN on the morning of the President's Commission announcement and my determination to chart a self-curing course as a plan blessed by God. It soon dawned on me for the first time that I was very likely deeply ensnared in the clutches of the opioid pain medications I was consuming. I had to seek answers if there were any to be found. Simultaneously,

Self-Cured Addict

I recognized, much like you, the inherent capability within us to navigate our way home from the challenges we encounter daily, even in unfamiliar territories. I believe this instinct is ingrained in the human soul—the yearning to attain God's blessing and freedom from addiction. And upon conquering your addiction, as I did, you will find Him watching and waiting for your triumphant return.

> *"Even the stork in the sky knows the seasons."*
> —*Jeremiah 8:7*

Individuals grappling with chronic pain resulting from surgical procedures or serious spinal and other injuries often find themselves susceptible to opioid use, addiction, abuse, or use disorders. Many, like myself, may remain unaware of their growing dependency and addiction, totally oblivious to the detrimental impact on their health of continuous opioid use. Consequently, they may not seek the advice of their physician for determining their need for specialized substance use treatment or referrals through to other more specialized practitioners. Barriers to seeking help as discussed previously often include issues of trust, reluctance to relinquish personal control to an unknown entity, limited options, financial constraints, inconvenient accessibility, lack of transportation, childcare needs, and long waiting lists.

Self-Cured Addict

"In all your ways acknowledge him, and he will make straight your path"
—*Proverbs 3:60*

Personally, I've always been averse to surrendering control to someone I don't know or trust. This certainly changed when I encountered incurable cancer but after more than eleven months of hospital control, I was ready to take back control over my future. When I made the decision to overcome my addiction, I chose to embark on researching how I could safely taper off the drugs under my own control. This led to the development of a comprehensive plan, process, and timeline. Early in my research, I discovered the severity of my addiction, realizing that the tapering process might extend over months or even a year. Armed with the knowledge acquired through my research, I felt empowered to take the necessary steps to formulate a long-term plan and initiate the tapering process. I did not know at the outset that the journey would result in inventing and patenting a barrier technology that would become FenBlock and its likely future family of similar products meant to address illicit narcotics. What I knew was that I had a choice. Did I choose the hell of drugs or to end my use of drugs? Perhaps you face a similar choice.

Self-Cured Addict

It is hard for me and I hope for you as well to imagine a more stupid or dangerous decision than putting decisions about me or you in the hands of people who pay no price for being wrong.

What I discovered is that millions of individuals who have been prescribed fentanyl and opioids are unaware of the associated health risks, and they are oblivious of the need to contemplate ending their use. While there is a significant emphasis on preventing opioid addiction and treating it through alternative medications or rehabilitation, I encountered a gap in methods specifically focused on curing addiction. Empowering the millions of Americans in need of a cure is crucial, and it is my hope that having information provided by me, a former opioid addict, will offer valuable substance and instill patient confidence.

I aim to serve as a credible resource, drawing from years of personal experience with fentanyl and opioid use and misuse that led to addiction, to help others better understand their reliance on opioids. It is essential for an individual to assess his or her level of addiction, abuse, or misuse and to take appropriate action. Subsequently involving a physician or medical provider as a coach, can significantly enhance the chances of successfully ending and curing an addiction.

Self-Cured Addict

We must rethink addiction's cure.

It's a problem that nobody has adequately addressed.

Throughout my seven years of opioid misuse and addiction, I observed that the health profession primarily focused on two fundamental areas: prevention and treatment. Approaches are general where I believe they need to be more focused on the specific types of opioids. The opioid problem most talked about is a product of a smaller feeder system of drug use—from gateway drugs such as marijuana being legalized to prescription opioids not having the proper physician oversight. As part of my research, I needed a unique solution for receiving lower, graduated dosages, particularly through a permeable transdermal patch applied to the patient's skin. Being a long-term user of fentanyl patches, I had to tackle the distinctiveness of the patch's design and develop a method for patients to gradually, through managed amounts, taper off fentanyl patches while minimizing the risks of misuse. The resulting graduating barrier technology invention, FenBlock, empowers individuals addicted to prescribed fentanyl patches, and potentially to other opioid medications and illicit drugs, to manage the tapering of those drugs, and with their physician's oversight and coaching, ultimately to completely cure their addiction. For example, under a physician's care, it may be possible to switch from pills or injected doses of opioids to a fentanyl patch. Then FenBlock can easily be employed to steadily reduce the dosage over time until freedom from addiction is achieved.

FenBlock[30] can mark the beginning of a new era in addressing cures for prescribed or illicit fentanyl and opioid addiction and use. This innovation is first of its kind. Its patented technology has the potential to offer a safe, user managed cure for other opioids, such as heroin and cocaine. My colleagues and I envision its future application will provide relief to addicted neonatal infants, ending their tragic and horrific withdrawal experiences. The successful development, validation, and market placement of this groundbreaking barrier would not be possible without the dedication, advice, and contributions of numerous individuals and organizations. As I articulate these advancements, our current focus includes seeking funding for the clinical validation of the FenBlock device, a crucial step toward its widespread implementation.

> *When a person is demoralized he cannot hear the truth.*
> *Don't let drugs demoralize you. Seek hope.*

In the pursuit of overcoming my addiction, I've reached out

to numerous politicians, ranging from the President of the United States to local state and national representatives, as well as cabinet secretaries. With the exception of the President, and my Congressman, unfortunately, my efforts have been met with silence, highlighting a common issue with politicians. Despite their public commitment to ending the opioid epidemic, they often engage in excessive talk without sufficient listening. This lack of responsiveness can be counterproductive to those searching for solutions, as the most effective approach to defeating addiction lies not just in convincing others of one's correctness but in demonstrating and highlighting genuine care about the subject. Politicians are attracted to the most published issues that resonate with their constituents. An example is their focus on cartel illicit fentanyl that they see as an easy target. Talk tough. Promise action. They miss the point that prescribed opioids and gateway drugs are feeders to many struggling with cartel-supplied illicit opioids. While their avoidance and silence has been disheartening, my unwavering personal resolve and faith-based purpose to move forward has been my most steadfast companion, helping me stay focused on my journey. You may assume you will face similar challenges. To that I say, stay strong, stay committed. You will achieve success. If I can help you, my contact information can be found at the back of the book. I will make myself available.

Self-Cured Addict

"Destiny doesn't make appointments. It usually shows up at the door unannounced. And it often knocks quietly, you have to listen carefully.[31]" Its quiet knock may be in this book.

Discovering the key to breaking free from addiction is like unlocking a hidden treasure. The secret lies in a simple yet profound principle: you receive by giving. Begin by acknowledging the blessings of seeking and achieving freedom from addiction. Then, transform these blessings into tangible rewards by extending a helping hand to others facing their own struggles with opioid addiction. Make this process a consistent part of your journey. In doing so, you'll find that destiny is not an external force but an inner strength waiting to be realized.

Chapter Six: Spreading the Word

*"I will instruct you and teach you in the way you should go;
I will counsel you with my eye upon you."*

—*Psalm 32: 8*

Following President Trump and Chris Christie's wake up call and my self cure, my goal was to take the process and the device I'd invented and used to end my addiction and bring them together to help others. I began by telling my story to whomever would listen and showing the device to whomever had an interest in seeing it. I began by writing letters to President and First Lady Trump. Then I wrote to every cabinet secretary and to Dr. Francis Collins, then the director of The National Institutes of Health. As you know from Part One, he quickly got in touch with me, and we spoke for forty minutes. Dr. Collins said that he was forwarding my letter to his deputy at the National Institute for Drug Abuse (NIDA) to let him know someone there should get in touch with me to discuss the process I'd developed and the device I had used to end my addiction.

The following week I received a call from NIDA. I was told that what I had developed was so unique that it was in need of protection, and that I should file a patent to both protect my idea (the process) and the device and that by doing so, it would indicate that I was serious in developing a medical device and service to help save the lives of others who face similar opioid dependency and addiction. NIDA became a mentor and we had numerous calls and exchanged numerous emails including a copy of my provisional patent.

During our many discussions I learned the NIDA policy limited their ability to respond to my request for assistance. The responsibility, for example, to locate a research team for possible clinical validation was to be mine alone, including identifying and contacting medical research centers where required validation could be performed. I was told NIDA would be available to answer questions and, where possible, to provide limited guidance, including how to locate addiction science medical research centers around the country. I also learned that if I wanted my idea to become a viable product, I needed to obtain the acceptance by a research center's Principal Investigators. Upon review, I was told that they might agree to establish a project to validate the process and medical device if they saw value in my process and invention. Through the research work, they would be then able to help attract a commercial partner and to determine market potential.

Self-Cured Addict

I began my search by searching for "opioid addiction research centers." From the results, I drilled into their websites and searched for "opioid." The results provided me with research center directors and the names and contact data for their independent investigators. For each one, I drafted a personal letter explaining my story of cancer and lengthy surgery and subsequent use and long term addiction to hydromorphone and fentanyl pain medications. In each letter I included a narrative description of the novel device FenBlock I'd invented and described how I'd used it in my successful tapering process. I also provided a description of my purpose, which of course was to "save the lives of other opioid addicted persons." I hoped this would capture their interest and lead to a means to bring the device to market.

I delved into how the process and novel device could liberate individuals from dependency or addiction to prescribed opioid / fentanyl pain medications and even illicit or street opioids. Emphasizing the benefit of patients having autonomy, I explored the two prevailing approaches to ending opioid use: substitution drugs and controlled withdrawal at rehabilitation centers. Motivated by my own quest for freedom from pain medication addiction, I explained that I had rejected both. Because I was uncertain of the extent of my dependency, I had been hesitant to relinquish control over my goal of ending my addiction. I underscored my concerns about potential mismanagement and the loss of agency in a rehabilitation program and noted the high rates of recidivism of both of the prevailing methods.

Regardless of the path one has tread to dependency or addiction, I believe that individuals should scrutinize their circumstances and employ my approach as a template for self-examination. While each journey may vary, the value of self-direction and empowerment is in my opinion paramount.

"Thanks to God that he gave me stubbornness when I know I am right."
— *John Adams*

My Team, and their impact

Here is something else you may find helpful. Upon my return home from the hospital, I took an initiative that yielded remarkable results, and I highly recommend you consider doing the same. I reached out to my local pharmacist and invited him to join my wife and me in monthly meetings with my personal physician. Our objective was to discuss my overall medication regimen, its impact on my daily health, and to address any potential concerns while making necessary adjustments in a timely manner. Having the support of a pain medication management team familiar with my condition might have been uncommon, and creative, yet it afforded me a deeper understanding and appreciation of potential interactions, including the risks associated with the prescribed opioid pain medication. I also believe the meetings were educational for all parties.

"Find no fear before your eyes. Draw upon faith and wisdom to patiently follow your path to freedom from addiction."

Addiction manifests itself through what I would describe as warning signals. These signs emerged during the tapering process. I categorized these indicators by measuring the reduction of frequency and intensity of headaches, nausea, depression, anxiety, sleep disturbances, and fluctuations in mood against my prior experiences with the same during the times of regular and increasing dosages.

"So intimately connected sometimes that it's unclear whether dependency on opioids should be addressed as one or many different opioid based drugs"

Self-Cured Addict

Throughout the graduated FenBlock tapering periods, all indicators continued to show positive results with no negative findings. Seeing this I was empowered to continue the process to its conclusion.

Chapter Seven: Overcoming Negativity

"Drug overdoses killed 63,632 Americans in 2016. Nearly two-thirds of these deaths (66%) involved a prescription or illicit opioid."[32]

Have you ever wished that overcoming addiction was as simple as just deciding to quit? Many have attempted to battle substance abuse by sheer willpower alone, only to find themselves returning to the cycle of addiction. The desire to reclaim freedom from harmful behaviors and to realize the vision of a brighter future can be strong, but it can be extremely challenging to actually bring it about. I know because I've had the experience and was able to find self empowerment through an established plan that allowed for tweaking and adjustment as it played out.

What if I told you that the most powerful tool for combating addiction resides within your own mind and heart? Addiction isn't merely a matter of behavioral patterns; it's a multifaceted disease rooted in the intricate workings of the brain's decision-making processes that may have been altered by powerful opioid drugs. Despite our best intentions, our brains can lead us astray, even as your heart reaches out

Self-Cured Addict

to God in an effort to compel you to engage in actions that will bring you hope, accomplishments, and success.

Keep your heart with all vigilance, for from
it flows the springs of life.
—Proverbs 4:23

The encouraging news is that by mastering the art of transforming negative thought patterns, you can reclaim authority over your life and conquer addiction. Embracing a mindset of positivity is a pivotal step on your journey to recovery, empowering you to cultivate resilience and resilience in the face of adversity. Like many others, my pursuit of a fulfilling my life was disrupted by addiction. Recognizing this, I embarked on a journey to reevaluate my values and principles, drawing the strength from them needed to overcome addiction and reclaim my freedom from drugs. These fundamental values and principles are accessible to us all, offering a powerful foundation for conquering addiction and embracing a fulfilling life once more.

My journey taught me that addiction doesn't discriminate; it affects us all equally, bringing about similar challenges and struggles. These difficulties often evoke feelings of unease and even embarrassment among those who grapple with it. The inevitable question arises, "Why me?" It's a fundamental query that cannot be ignored.

I found the structural barriers previously discussed, such as limited access to treatment, healthcare disparities, and criminalization of drug use, which hindered my recovery efforts. I pray my story will inspire hope and demonstrate that recovery from fentanyl / opioid addiction and use is possible. Despite the dignity that addiction attempted to strip away from, I resolved to take proactive steps towards recovery, cherishing each new day as a gift. You can do the same.

Taking charge of your situation and embracing the challenges that will likely be encountered ahead will allow you to adopt a mindset of resilience. Understood that the journey to recovery will likely not be linear. There will be ups and downs along the way. Despite the uncertainties, you must remain committed to your tapering plan and acknowledge that the progress may not always be straightforward. Expect to encounter some discomfort, and emotional turmoil, and adjust your approach if necessary based on your evolving needs and experiences.

When we stop fearing failure only then can we seize opportunity.

Self-Cured Addict

Drawing from my own journey of opioid addiction and tapering, I highly recommend considering the FenBlock method if you're contemplating tapering from a fentanyl patch. As you certainly know by now, at this writing the device is working its way through the FDA. The approach offers a safe, straightforward, and effective self-managed solution to overcoming addiction. Just as it worked for me, I am confident it will work for you as you set your goals and navigate your tapering journey towards freedom from addiction.

Remember that the scripture says, *"And behold, I am with you always, until the end of the age"* (Matthew 28:20). This message resonates deeply with me, reminding me of the constant presence of support and guidance even in the darkest moments of addiction and the fight against its surrounding stigma; the ignorant judgment by others.

When I speak of things getting better, it's not a dismissal of the harsh realities of addiction that exist both in my world and yours. Even after months and years of being free from fentanyl, and all opioids, I remain committed to sharing my story with those in prisons, health officials, our native American tribes and nations, schools, and recovery centers. I want to shed light on the challenges of addiction. However, I also believe in the power of progress and the possibility of transformation. Embracing your journey towards ending fentanyl or any opioid dependency is a noble endeavor, a step towards a more fulfilling life. Think of your addiction as a premature baby in an incubator. Consider the baby's health status at the beginning of their life like your opioid dependency. It can be extremely bad at the beginning. Breathing, heart rate, and other important signs from opioid use should be tracked constantly so that changes for better or worse can be seen, quickly. After a week, the baby will be getting a lot better. During your first week of tapering, you may not recognize a difference. On all the main measurement points, the baby will be improving, but it has to stay in the incubator because its health remains critical. For you, too, are improving while you keep yourself on a near normal schedule of [reduced] opioid dosages. Slowly, you continue tapering through a graduated barrier technique like FenBlock from your normal dosages to greater and greater amounts—finally to the point of ending your use and addiction. Each step should be recorded in a daily log that should include a description of all side effects. You will want to share the log and your notes with your physician at each appointment.

If your dream of Freedom from Addiction doesn't scare you, it's too small.

Does it make sense to suggest that both the infant's and your situation are improving? Absolutely. Does it also make sense to acknowledge that the situation may still have challenges? Absolutely. Does stating "things are improving" imply that all is well and we should relax? No. Is it helpful to feel compelled to categorize situations as either bad or improving? Certainly not. It's both. It's both challenging and improving. Never feel disheartened by the amount of time it takes for improvement to unfold. It's a mixture of progress and [temporary] setbacks, happening simultaneously, and it's all under your control.

The beauty lies in having the autonomy to set your own timeline for improvement, just as I was able to do. We possess the power to choose the pace and method to end our use through tapering. Unlike the baby, we can follow a process that empowers us to continue the journey towards freedom from addiction while recognizing the current realities. It's our responsibility to navigate this journey by exerting control over our actions.

This mindset reflects optimism within us. We see the glass as half full, not half empty. These truths guide our internal reflections and understanding of our condition. We hold firm to the belief that we are attaining freedom from addiction. This is the perspective we must maintain. There's no need to anticipate perfection; it's the journey that matters.

"I can do all things through Him who strengthens me."
—Ph 4:13

In times of uncertainty, it is essential to remain patient and to be adaptable, ready to adjust goals and timelines as needed. If doubts arise, as they often do, seeking guidance through prayer can offer clarity and direction. Discuss any concerns and uncertainties with your physician. I've found that my faith has been a guiding light, in decisions and in discussions with my physician, family and friends. They all provided opinions and answers and kept me aligned with my objectives, even during challenging moments.

May you be open to the search for all that is true to give you strength and persuasion when needed.

As we move ahead together, I will do my best to give insight concerning how to navigate the challenges of overcoming fentanyl / opioid use addiction. Remember to draw upon your faith first. It is where you will find your inner courage and resilience. Our paths forward may be uncertain, and there may be moments of discomfort as you work towards ending your use. It's important to acknowledge within reason that reducing dosages can lead to increased pain levels, which may vary in intensity and timing for every individual. Long-term opioid use can also result, as it did in my case, in the accumulation of opiates in your body's tissues, causing a delayed response to tapering efforts. So be prepared to accept and adjust your timeline. There is nothing wrong or weak in adjusting as long as your target remains in sight.

Draw upon your courage and tap into inner strengths and resources as you face challenges and overcome obstacles. Take bold actions. Here are a few tips I used that you may find useful:

Acknowledge Your Uncertainty, Your Fear: Recognize that feeling of doubt and fear is natural and normal. Instead of trying to suppress or ignore it, acknowledge your doubt or fear and understand that courage is within you. It is not the absence of fear but the ability to act despite it. This must be a continual part of your journey. I understood my many uncertainties. We all experience them from time to time. But I always remembered my source of strength through re-reading Proverbs 3:5-6 "Trust in the Lord with all your heart, and do not lean on your own understanding.

In all your ways acknowledge him, and he will make your path straight."

Identify Your Values: Clarify and prioritize what matters most to you and what you stand for. When you align your faith, actions with your values, you can find the motivation and determination to face difficult situations with courage. I reminded myself of the voice of God as He said to us all in Isaiah 43:2, "When you pass through the waters, I will be with you; and through the rivers, they shall not overwhelm you; when you walk through fire you shall not be burned, and the flame shall not consume you."

Set Clear Goals: Clearly define what you want to achieve and why it's important to you. I even prioritized my list to provide further clarity for myself. Having a clear sense of purpose, your mission, can provide the motivation and focus needed to overcome obstacles and stay committed to your goals, even when things get tough.

Practice Self-Compassion: Be kind and gentle with yourself, especially when facing challenges or setbacks. Treat yourself with the same compassion and understanding that you would offer to a friend in a similar situation. 1 Peter 3:8 brings us the needed understanding of compassion that is so important to our success. "Finally, all of you, have unity of mind, sympathy, brotherly love, a tender heart, and a humble mind."

Take Incremental Steps: Work, discuss your concerns and seek suggested steps with your physician as I did in order to break down what may appear to be daunting tasks into smaller, more manageable steps. By taking smaller, more achievable actions towards your goals, you can build confidence and momentum over time, gradually expanding your comfort zone and strengthening your courage muscle.

Seek Support: Surround yourself with supportive people who believe in you and encourage you to be your best self. Lean on friends, family, mentors, or support groups for guidance, encouragement, and perspective when facing challenges. I found this to be one of the most beneficial steps throughout my months of graduated tapering. Their support was incredible.

Reflect on Past Successes: Remind yourself by reaching back to your daily log of the times when you've demonstrated courage and overcome challenges. Reflecting on your past successes can boost your confidence and they will remind you of your ability to overcome adversity.

By incorporating these strategies into your life and by building your plan to end your use of opioids / fentanyl, you can cultivate the courage needed to tackle challenges, pursue your goals, and live through your faith in alignment with your values.

To mitigate uncertainties and physical effects, prioritize staying hydrated and prepare for potential withdrawal symptoms while tapering. Understand that there may be moments of discouragement along the way, but know that you possess the internal strength and determination to persevere. With unwavering commitment and solidarity to your journey, success will be reached.

> *"No temptation has overtaken you except what is common to mankind."*
> —*1-Cor 10:13-14*

I examined the significant challenges and found it beneficial to apply the 80/20 rule. Allow me to explain. Often, we assume that all challenges carry equal weight, yet in reality, only a few are paramount compared to the rest, even when they are combined. For instance, when faced with the task of tapering multiple opioids, the crucial question arises: which opioid should be the starting point?

Self-Cured Addict

Focusing on identifying the challenges that constituted eighty percent of the total, I was able to prioritize effectively. It is also important to align challenges with available resources such as time and energy. Before dedicating efforts to smaller tasks, it's essential to identify and rank the core challenges: why they are significant and what implications they hold. This approach proved effective for me as it kept me focused on the pivotal milestones and minimized distractions as I moved ahead.

You, too, can adopt this strategy. Despite initially planning for a timeframe of ten to eleven months, I discovered that in reality, it took fourteen months to successfully overcome my opioid addiction. The sense of accomplishment I derived from the journey remains palpable. In essence, empowering yourself to tackle challenges head-on is key to achieving significant feats.

Support Groups

In addition to the strategy and tactics discussed above, it may also be beneficial to seek out support from others, and numerous support groups exist outside family and friends, offering a range of supportive treatments (not cures) for opioid addiction within most communities. Among the more common groups are Narcotics Anonymous and Opiates Anonymous. Both are known to provide assistance to those struggling with addiction. While locating an Opiates Anonymous group may prove challenging, there are typically numerous Narcotics Anonymous groups in each state, providing support to individuals ready to quit. However, my personal experience with Narcotics Anonymous was underwhelming and reinforced my decision to self-manage my tapering process. If you are blessed with a network of supportive family and friends, my suggestion is to team up with them along with your physician. If you are unable to have such a support structure I recommend initiating an inquiry through the local group's website for more information.

Suffering with addiction produced endurance that strengthened my character. Through strong character came hope that put all doubters to shame.

As you view support groups it is essential to understand no one who has ever lived has failed to experience conflicts between reason and emotion; the difference is between the person who has weak self command or who lacks the character trait required to discipline desire.

Self-Cured Addict

One of the notable concerns I observed about treatment centers and support groups is the inclination that seems to exist in them to impose replacement therapy or rehabilitative therapy as a way to address addiction without considering the deep concern a patient might have about the pain and withdrawal symptons that are likely to come about as a result. While the methods of replacement therapy may vary slightly from one medication to another, the underlying concept is straightforward: Administer a medication that signals the body to believe it is receiving opiates, thereby mitigating withdrawal symptoms and facilitating the detox process. However, my assessment led me to conclude that the majority of these centers prioritize revenue generation and focus more on addressing illicit or street opiates rather than prescribed addiction. As a patient grappling with prescription addiction, I found myself in captive will, and I sought to break the captive role drugs were playing. To that end I tried to find support from individuals who could directly relate to my challenges, and yet I found this level of understanding lacking in my search. As I deliberated and found support to further influence me I did not want to fail to abide by my decision. It's important to exercise caution as you deliberate, commit, and enact your mission and pathway and as you interact with local groups that may refer you to their resources.

Here are some of the replacement therapy medications commonly encountered if you opt for this route. However, it's crucial to note that these medications are addictive as well:

Methadone: Widely used for replacing heroin or other opiates to alleviate withdrawal symptoms associated with opiate detox. Methadone is highly addictive and its use as a medication replacement should be closely monitored by a physician. Personally, I prefer therapy centers that prioritize discussions on long-term cure rather than detox, but preferences may vary among individuals.

Suboxone: A relatively new method of medical replacement therapy deemed highly effective in aiding patients in overcoming opiate addiction. Suboxone has the tendency to induce sickness if opioids are used while under treatment with this medication. In my personal experience, following the process I laid out for myself resulted in no instances of nausea, unlike the daily and intense nausea caused by the opioids I was prescribed.

Naltrexone: This medication blocks the euphoric and sedative effects of opiates and is known to reduce opiate cravings. Naltrexone is commonly used as part of maintenance therapy to help patients stay sober and prevent relapse, as it inhibits feelings of euphoria and may induce sudden and severe withdrawal symptoms. With the right timeline and dosage management tailored to your comfort level, withdrawal symptoms can be minimized, and the need for a medical solution like naltrexone may not be warranted as was the case for me.

Regardless of therapy we must hold ourselves and the other clinicians involved in our care accountable. If we are to develop effective treatment strategies for persons like me and maybe you with prescribed or illicit substance use disorders, we must understand that these patients cover an entire spectrum, ranging from those whose abstinence is considerably related to personal responsibility, to those whose abstinence will require intensive psychiatric and rehabilitative treatment. I found myself to be a responsible person who studied and understood the path to freedom of use. However, if you recognize that you are having problems understanding the pathway and have difficulty exercising free will, then you need to seek help to become stronger along with someone to mentor your pathway in order to achieve success.

No document previously published says so much and provides proactive guidance as the medical device (FenBlock) that brings triumph over opioid addiction.

Self-Cured Addict

The statement above encapsulates the rationale behind my decision to seize control of my addiction to substantial doses of fentanyl and hydromorphone. My reflections on the existing practices for detoxification and tapering are intended to bolster your endeavors to break free from addiction. Moreover, I trust that sharing my story will inspire and empower you on your journey towards liberation from opioid and other addictive drugs.

Chapter Eight: The Need for a Fentanyl / Opioid Czar

Why the End Justifies a New Means

The United States' fentanyl crisis is expanding at a time when it should be going in the other direction as the result of government and stakeholder focused resources and efforts. At N Brereton Medical Technologies we see the need to reverse the trend and have based our research and development on the nation's need to adopt a new strategic focus, rather than continue the processes as we see them today. Our belief is a more teleological approach will lead to more innovative and effective solutions, such as Fen-Block™, in addressing the complex issues surrounding fentanyl use and addiction.

The teleological imperative for government intervention in the fentanyl and addiction crisis is clear: to preserve life, alleviate suffering, and restore societal stability. This crisis not only claims lives through misuse or overdose, but it also fractures communities, burdens healthcare systems, and strains law enforcement resources. Therefore, the government's role should be driven by a consistent, purpose-focused approach that prioritizes and enforces positive outcomes.

Self-Cured Addict

Governments are uniquely positioned to marshal resources, legislate effective policies, and implement comprehensive strategies that can address the multifaceted dimensions of this epidemic. By focusing on the end goal of reducing the human and societal toll of addiction, policy measures can be designed to maximize compliance enforcement effectiveness and efficiency. This includes increasing access to life-saving interventions like naloxone and FenBlock, enhancing public health monitoring, supporting evidence-based treatment modalities, and addressing underlying socioeconomic and medical prescription practices that inadvertently contribute to the opioid and fentanyl addiction crisis. We see our government's need to better understand these factors as critical for healthcare providers, policymakers, and the public to help uniformly mitigate risks and manage prescribed medication appropriately while reducing the potential for abuse.

In fulfilling this teleological need, the government must not only act but do so homogeneously and ethically, with a commitment to the dignity and worth of every individual affected by this crisis. Today the government acts disparately. The measures adopted should be uniformly evaluated not just on their intent or the resources expended but on their actual impact in alleviating the crisis and improving public health. This need for an improved focused and outcome-based approach is not merely an administrative responsibility, but a moral duty to protect and enhance the lives of citizens, demonstrating the government's fundamental role in safeguarding the welfare of its people.

The current landscape of fentanyl / opioid control and enforcement in the United States is characterized by a patchwork of strategies and policies that vary widely across states and agencies. This lack of uniformity has led to significant inefficiencies and inconsistencies in addressing one of the most critical public health crises of our time—the opioid and fentanyl epidemic. The disparate nature of these efforts not only hampers the effectiveness of interventions but also complicates the ability to implement comprehensive, coordinated responses and to encourage innovative solutions.

We must as a nation demand the establishment of a Fentanyl/Opioid Czar within the administration as a crucial step toward rectifying these inconsistencies and shortcomings. A central authority would provide the unified leadership necessary to streamline efforts across federal, state, and local levels. With a singular focus on the fentanyl / opioid crisis, the Czar could ensure that resources are allocated efficiently, policies are consistent and grounded in the latest scientific research, and that there is accountability in achieving measurable goals.

Moreover, a Czar could foster greater collaboration among law enforcement, healthcare providers, public health officials, entrepreneurs, and community organizations, creating a more integrated approach to prevention, treatment, recovery, and enforcement. The role would also facilitate more effective data collection and analysis, allowing for innovation, invention and rapid adaptation of technologies and strategies in response to emerging trends and evidence.

The creation of a Fentanyl / Opioid Czar position would not merely be an administrative change but a necessary fundamental shift towards a more strategic and coordinated battle against the epidemic. By centralizing command and focusing our national efforts, we will better be able to protect public health, reduce the burden on healthcare and criminal justice systems, and most importantly, save lives. The establishment of a dedicated Fentanyl and Opioid Czar within the government is a teleologically driven initiative step, rooted in the purposeful and urgent need to address the burgeoning fentanyl / opioid crisis with effective leadership and coordinated action. The role of a Fentanyl and Opioid Czar will serve a clear end goal: